D1246932

DR. COLBERT'S HEALTHY BRAIN ZONE

DON COLBERT, MD

SILOAM

Most Charisma Media products are available at special quantity discounts for bulk purchase for sales promotions, premiums, fund-raising, and educational needs. For details, call us at (407) 333-0600 or visit our website at www.charismamedia.com.

Dr. Colbert's Healthy Brain Zone by Don Colbert, MD
Published by Siloam, an imprint of Charisma Media
600 Rinehart Road, Lake Mary, Florida 32746

Visit the author's website at drcolbert.com, www.drcolbertbooks.com.

Cataloging-in-Publication Data is on file with the Library of Congress.
International Standard Book Number: 978-1-63641-109-5
E-book ISBN: 978-1-63641-110-1

This book contains the opinions and ideas of its author. It is solely for informational and educational purposes and should not be regarded as a substitute for professional medical treatment. The nature of your body's health condition is complex and unique. Therefore, you should consult a health professional before you begin any new exercise, nutrition, or supplementation program or if you have questions about your health. Neither the author nor the publisher shall be liable or responsible for any loss or damage allegedly arising from any information or suggestion in this book.

People and names in this book are composites created by the author from his experiences as a medical doctor. Names and details of their stories have been changed, and any similarity between the names and stories of individuals described in this book and individuals known to readers is purely coincidental.

The statements in this book about consumable products or food have not been evaluated by the Food and Drug Administration. The recipes in this book are to be followed exactly as written. The publisher is not responsible for your specific health or allergy needs that may require medical supervision. The publisher is not responsible for any adverse reactions to the consumption of food or products that have been suggested in this book.

While the author has made every effort to provide accurate internet addresses at the time of publication, neither the publisher nor the author assumes any responsibility for errors or for changes that occur after publication. Further, the publisher does not have any control over and does not assume any responsibility for author or third-party websites or their content.

23 24 25 26 27 — 987654321
Printed in the United States of America

For God has not given us a spirit of fear,
but of power and of love and of a sound mind.
—2 Timothy 1:7

DEDICATION

THIS BOOK IS dedicated to my mother, Kitty Colbert, and my father, Don Colbert Sr., who both battled Alzheimer's disease. My father died of Alzheimer's disease and pneumonia at age eighty.

He started having mild memory problems and confusion in his mid- to late forties. My sister and I remember when he drove us to the University of Mississippi and other towns in Mississippi and how he would become confused with directions and get turned around.

In his fifties he became even more confused as his memory deteriorated. Once he visited my home when I was newly married, and he tried to organize my garage and my house, but he stacked boxes and stuff in a corner, with the boxes too high, where they could all topple over. It was disorganized and haphazard.

He then started layering his clothing and would ask the same questions repeatedly. His memory worsened in his sixties, and my mother put him in a daytime Alzheimer's care center. He then became paranoid and would hide things from my mother, including money and valuables.

By seventy he had to be admitted to a full-time Alzheimer's care facility. In his seventies he lost most of his communication skills, but he still loved to sing and whistle. My father's amazing ability to whistle beautifully was one of the last functions he lost.

He would love it when my brother, Dan, would come to the nursing home and play the piano. My father would sing and rock back and forth on his heels as he sang with all his heart. He especially loved the old hymns.

His condition continued to deteriorate, and eventually he could not communicate at all. Shortly before he died, I introduced my then infant grandson, Braden, to his great-grandfather. My father's eyes lit up initially but then went back to their blank stare. He didn't comprehend who Braden was.

Shortly after that, he died of pneumonia. That was in 2009, and I had been searching for years for the answers, but there was no medicine or combination of medications that would stop the progression of Alzheimer's.

Since that time, Dale Bredesen, MD, a world-renowned neurologist, has found that Alzheimer's disease can be prevented and, in many cases, reversed if diagnosed and treated soon enough. He claims there are thirty-six metabolic factors that, if imbalanced, can trigger downsizing of the brain.

My mother developed mild dementia a few years ago that is most likely due to type 2 diabetes, which she has had for more than thirty years. She worked full time at a bank until she was eighty-two. Her brain was very sharp.

I started her on a good nutritional program years ago, and even though she has a sweet tooth and still eats some sugar, the program has improved her condition dramatically. She had some setbacks or temporary worsening of her memory, such as when she had hip surgery and received general anesthesia and again when she had COVID-19. However, I was able to give her the appropriate supplements that got her through these issues. My mother is now eighty-seven years old and going strong. She is not lacking for any conversation.

I pray this book will give you the road map to protect your brain or slow, manage, stop, or reverse Alzheimer's and dementia.

CONTENTS

PREFACE

YOU NEED TO know that Alzheimer's and dementia do not have to be the end of the road. Also, because there is an amyloid precursor protein (APP) "switch" that turns these diseases on, it stands to reason that there is an APP switch that turns them off. (Read more on APP in chapter 4.) Here are some positive things to keep in mind as you read this book:

- Just as things progress downward, things can turn around and progress upward.
- Symptoms that show up can many times be reversed and go away.
- Ground that has been lost can usually be gained back.

I've seen all this and more happen with hundreds of my patients. Patients with mild to moderate Alzheimer's and dementia have improved, gotten their jobs back, driven again, and even been "in remission" with the disease. And even patients with severe Alzheimer's and dementia have seen improvement in their memory and health.

In the pages that follow, you will find a proven and effective pathway to many times fix the underlying problems that cause Alzheimer's and dementia. The best course of action is always preventive, and the second-best is treating it immediately. Don't wait until next year.

Bottom line: there is hope, which is something we all need.

—DON COLBERT, MD

PART I: WHAT'S GOING ON?

PEOPLE RECOIL WHEN the word *Alzheimer's* or *dementia* is used. They step back, and usually fear grips their hearts as well as their minds! But despite the rampant trends, news, or statistics, there is hope! There are answers out there. No magic pill makes everything go away, but proven steps, protocols, health measures, and options can truly help slow, manage, stop, or reverse Alzheimer's and dementia. If you are on this journey for yourself or friends or family, I encourage you not to delay. Time is of the essence, so jump in right away and apply all that you learn.

CHAPTER 1

WHY THE EXPLOSION OF ALZHEIMER'S AND DEMENTIA?

FIRST THINGS FIRST: You need to know that Alzheimer's and dementia are not diseases or sicknesses that you *catch*. Nor do they suddenly, randomly, unexpectedly appear. Rather, Alzheimer's and dementia are the body's responses to what we are feeding it, doing to it, not giving it, and exposing it to, and all around how we are mistreating it. The body and brain are simply trying to cope.

Sadly, millions of people around the world are knowingly and unknowingly mistreating their brains on a daily basis. An explosive wave of resulting Alzheimer's and dementia cases will devastate lives, families, communities, businesses, and nations. And it's all unnecessary. It doesn't have to happen, which means you can usually stop it if it's diagnosed soon enough and appropriate action is taken.

GLOBAL EXPLOSION

I can tell you exactly where Alzheimer's and dementia cases currently rank: right behind the obesity epidemic wave. Today, more than 40 percent of American adults are obese (having a body mass index greater than or equal to 30), which is up from only 13 percent in the 1960s. The number of overweight and obese people has never been this high, and it's only getting higher![1]

Our children are following our example. In the last thirty years alone, obesity in children has doubled, and in adolescents it has tripled.[2]

Alzheimer's and dementia cases are also right behind the type 2 diabetes epidemic wave. According to the Centers for Disease Control and

Prevention (CDC), in 1976 only five million Americans had diabetes.[3] Today, more than one hundred million are diabetic or have prediabetes.[4]

That is not all.

It's not just one big wave, one explosion, or one cause. There are many waves. Alzheimer's and dementia are coming, wave after wave, crashing on our shores, destroying far more than we could have ever imagined.

The fact that there are many waves of Alzheimer's and dementia makes good sense because people seldom have just one type of Alzheimer's.[5] They usually have two or more types of Alzheimer's when they are finally diagnosed.

Each wave of Alzheimer's and dementia follows a different cause. Yes, it follows right behind obesity and type 2 diabetes, but it also usually follows behind other things, such as

- chronic inflammation,
- chronic stress,
- exposure to toxins,
- general anesthesia,
- genetics,
- gum disease,
- insulin resistance,
- a lack of key nutrients,
- a leaky gut,
- low oxygen while sleeping,
- a poor diet, including bad fats,
- a sedentary lifestyle,
- unbalanced hormones,
- and more!

IT'S A FACT

Women are twice as likely as men to get Alzheimer's or dementia.[6]

The number of people with Alzheimer's and dementia is expected to triple in the next thirty years. It's already the third-costliest disease in the United States, with more than one hundred billion dollars spent annually.[7] Is that a bill that families can pick up?

Alzheimer's and dementia cases are hitting every country. Without changing the paradigm, without making changes at the personal level, and without doing something different from the masses, the statistics will only continue to rise.

Thankfully, there are answers. There is something you can do about it. You do not need to accept the status quo, the age-related "normal," or the genetic history you may have inherited.

The waves need not overcome you.

CHAPTER 2

WHAT EXACTLY ARE ALZHEIMER'S AND DEMENTIA?

DEMENTIA HAS BEEN known and studied for hundreds of years. The term was first used around AD 600. In Latin it means "a state out of mind."[1] Aptly named, several different types of dementia were known to exist.

Alzheimer's disease would have been considered a type of dementia, but it wasn't until the early 1900s that it got its name. In 1901, Alois Alzheimer, a German doctor who studied psychiatry and neuropathology, was working at a mental hospital when Auguste Deter was admitted. She was fifty-one years old but acted as if she had advanced dementia.

Her symptoms included memory loss, delusions, disorientation, manic episodes, insomnia, and severe agitation. She could no longer work, manage the home, cook, or communicate rationally.

Dr. Alzheimer studied her symptoms as he worked with her. The mental hospital did its best to care for her, but not much could be done besides keeping her fed, clothed, and safe.

When she died in 1906 of septicemia and pneumonia, Dr. Alzheimer performed a biopsy of her brain. What he found—amyloid plaque and neurofibrillary tangles—are the same things we find today in Alzheimer's patients.[2] They are the telltale signs of the disease.

IT'S NOT A SINGLE DISEASE

Many people use *Alzheimer's* and *dementia* interchangeably, but this is inaccurate. There are four types of dementia, and Alzheimer's is one of them. And there are five types of Alzheimer's. Clearly this is not about a single disease wreaking havoc.

Types of dementia

Here is how it breaks down for the dementias:

1. Alzheimer's disease (70 percent of dementia cases)
2. Lewy body dementia (20 percent of dementia cases)
3. Vascular dementia (this type and type 4 make up the remaining 10 percent of dementia cases)
4. Frontotemporal dementia (also called Pick's disease)

Alzheimer's disease is marked by the well-known signs of amyloid plaque and neurofibrillary tangles in the brain, primarily in the brain's temporal lobes. Though these plaques and tangles are present, they do not cause Alzheimer's.

Symptoms of Lewy body dementia include delusions, hallucinations, and flailing about while sleeping. This type of dementia is more common among those with Parkinson's disease. Vascular dementia is typified by many small strokes. Frontotemporal dementia is associated with significant difficulty speaking and comprehending speech (aphasia) and inappropriate or compulsive behavior in social situations. It usually affects personality before it affects memory and is associated with unexpected mood changes. Picks disease usually starts between the ages of forty to sixty, with the average being age fifty-four.[3]

All dementias include memory problems. Only vascular dementia has known causes: a lack of blood flow to the brain, strokes, ministrokes (TIAs), and brain bleeds, usually due to vascular disease.

As you can see by these short descriptions, it is very easy for people to have many different symptoms of different types of dementia simultaneously. One or more of these dementias may coexist, which has been known to cause confusion when diagnosing patients.

Types of Alzheimer's disease

As for Alzheimer's disease and its five different types, here is how it breaks down:

1. Type 1 Alzheimer's (inflammatory or hot)

2. *Type 1.5 Alzheimer's (glycotoxic or sweet)*
3. Type 2 Alzheimer's (atrophic or cold)
4. Type 3 Alzheimer's (toxic or vile)
5. Type 4 Alzheimer's (vascular or pale)
6. Type 5 Alzheimer's (traumatic or dazed)[4]

You'll notice I've added a sixth type (type 1.5) because it is the most common among my patients. It is a mixture of types 1 and 2 and follows chronic inflammation and high insulin levels. If your hemoglobin A1c, blood sugar, and fasting insulin levels are elevated, your Alzheimer's chances increase. It's been said that about 40 percent of Americans are now insulin resistant.[5] That means they have glucose toxicity, which ages the brain rapidly. No wonder obesity and type 2 diabetes are followed closely by this type of Alzheimer's disease.

IT'S A FACT

Mainstream medicine assumes Alzheimer's is a single disease, but it's not.

Type 1 Alzheimer's follows chronic, ongoing inflammation. The effect of nonstop chronic inflammation is incredibly dangerous. Chronic inflammation is at the core of almost all chronic diseases, which includes Alzheimer's, along with most cancers, Parkinson's disease, cardiovascular disease, arthritis, autoimmune disease (rheumatoid arthritis, lupus, multiple sclerosis, colitis, Crohn's disease), and many more. Type 1 Alzheimer's is usually associated with elevated inflammatory markers, including an elevated C-reactive protein, an increase in tumor necrosis factor, an increase in interleukin-6 (IL-6), or an increase in nuclear factor kappa B (NFKB). It is also associated with a decrease in the albumin-to-globulin ratio. In other words, the albumin-to-globulin ratio decreases with excessive inflammation.[6]

Trust me when I say that you don't want long-term inflammation in your body because you are inviting Type 1 Alzheimer's disease into your brain.

Type 2 Alzheimer's follows those with suboptimal or low levels of sex, adrenal, and thyroid hormones, nutrients, and nerve cell growth factors, such as nerve growth factor (NGF) and brain-derived neurotrophic factor (BDNF). These levels can be remedied with the right supplements and bioidentical hormones, which may remove the symptoms entirely. Vitamin D levels are usually low or low normal. Homocysteine levels are usually elevated, and hormone levels (especially DHEA, pregnenolone, total and free testosterone, estradiol, progesterone, and thyroid hormone free T3) are usually low or low normal.[7]

Type 3 Alzheimer's follows exposure to toxins, be it from food, occupation, mold, soil, water, or other sources, such as mercury, lead, arsenic, cadmium, and excess copper. Toxic buildup from heavy metals can lead in this direction. The symptoms will only continue without removing the source of the toxins and then the toxins themselves.

IT'S A FACT

"Alzheimer's disease is actually a protective response of the brain to…different insults: microbes and other inflammagens, insulin resistance, toxins, and the loss of support by nutrients, hormones, growth factors. It is a protective downsizing program."[8]

Type 4 Alzheimer's follows cardiovascular disease, plaque buildup, and poor blood flow in the arteries to the brain. With heart disease being the number one killer in the world,[9] a lot of people are at risk for this dementia type. High blood pressure, smoking, diabetes, and high cholesterol levels can also increase the risk of vascular dementia.

Type 5 Alzheimer's follows head trauma (concussions), whether major or minor repeated head injuries. Younger people have less risk, but head trauma can accelerate Alzheimer's symptoms for those over age fifty. If you have the ApoE4 gene (the gene associated with Alzheimer's), a moderate head injury increases the risk of developing Alzheimer's disease tenfold.[10]

With all forms of Alzheimer's and dementia, brain cells and synapses (brain cell connections) degenerate and eventually die as amyloid plaques and tangles accumulate and destroy brain cells and synapses. It is a downsizing of the brain due to multiple factors, including chronic inflammation; a deficiency of key hormones, nutrients, and brain nutrients; progressive insulin resistance of brain cells; and glycation of the brain from a diet high in sugar, carbs, and starches. Also, toxic exposure from any of the ten or more dementogens I'll introduce in coming chapters can accelerate the downsizing of the brain. When the brain shuts down those areas of the brain that are clogged with amyloid plaques and tangles, the brain is trying to protect itself. It's the body's downsizing program for the brain.[11] Obviously, you don't want those plaques and tangles in your brain because you don't want those areas to shut down!

What Alzheimer's and Dementia Are to You

The amazing news is that Alzheimer's and dementia are hurdles that most people can overcome if caught soon enough. Speed bumps, if you will. Today they are usually not roadblocks that mark the end of the road, as they were in the past. Whatever memory loss or type of dementia you or a loved one might have been diagnosed with, there are effective answers today that Dr. Alzheimer never had at his disposal.

As you already know, Alzheimer's and dementia result from a body trying to cope with its environment. Change the environment and give the brain the nutrients, hormones, and growth factors that it needs, and Alzheimer's and dementia symptoms will usually improve—and sometimes disappear, if addressed soon enough.

To you, Alzheimer's and dementia are speed bumps. You can usually roll right over them.

CHAPTER 3

HOW DO YOU KNOW IF YOU HAVE IT?

Because you cannot catch Alzheimer's, the typical way someone begins to wonder if they have it is by looking for signs that gradually worsen over time. That is why all memory-related issues are divided into three stages: mild, moderate, and severe.

Most people who are diagnosed with Alzheimer's disease have experienced (and perhaps ignored) symptoms for ten, fifteen, or twenty years before their diagnosis. They didn't suddenly get it; they already had it, and it progressively worsened over time.

As I mentioned in chapter 2, Alzheimer's is the most common dementia. The following list is a standard breakdown of what happens at each stage of Alzheimer's if its progress goes unchecked.

Keep in mind that people with mild and moderate Alzheimer's disease (and all dementias) can usually expect to recover if they take the necessary steps. I have even had many patients on the border between moderate and severe who have made incredible turnarounds.

For those in the severe stages of Alzheimer's or other dementias, much can be done to help, slow, manage, stop, and sometimes improve memory loss, especially following the protocol explained in this book.

The time is always now to act. If you or your loved ones are around age fifty, that is the time when preventive action will bring you the most benefit. You may need to play a little catch-up if you are older, but it's great that you are starting now.

Regardless of your age, if you already have some signs of memory-related illness, then start right away. It's not common, but I have had patients in their thirties and forties whose brains looked more like those of a sixty- or seventy-year-old person. Thankfully, we were able to take action, and they were able to reclaim their lives, reverse the symptoms, and move on. Again, with the brain, earlier is always better.

Mild cognitive impairment (MCI) is an early stage of memory loss in individuals who can still live independently and carry out most activities of daily living. MCI may be the beginning stages of dementia. However, not everyone with MCI will develop dementia or Alzheimer's disease. MCI usually causes mild, unnoticeable deterioration of memory. People with MCI can still manage their daily activities and can still drive. About 10–20 percent of people sixty-five and older have MCI.[1]

Here are the typical signs of Alzheimer's disease at each stage, according to the Alzheimer's Association.

Mild

- Having difficulty performing tasks in a social or work setting
- Forgetting material that you just read
- Experiencing increased trouble with planning or organizing
- Losing or misplacing objects or documents
- Having trouble remembering names of new people
- Struggling to find the right word

Moderate

- Experiencing changes in sleep patterns
- Being confused about where you are or what day it is
- Feeling moody or withdrawn, especially in socially or mentally challenging situations
- Forgetting events or part of personal history
- Getting lost
- Needing help choosing appropriate clothes for day or event
- Having personality or behavior changes
- Experiencing suspiciousness, delusions, or compulsive behaviors
- Having trouble controlling bladder or bowels
- Being unable to remember own address or phone number, high school, or college

- Wandering

Severe

- Forgetting surroundings
- Having increased difficulty communicating
- Losing basic physical abilities: walking, sitting, or swallowing
- Having low awareness of recent happenings
- Needing 24-7 care
- Having vulnerability to infections, especially pneumonia[2]

If you think you have cognitive decline, the time to start reversing it is now. Doctors commonly tell patients, "Let's see how you are next year when you come back for your next checkup." I say, "Do not wait until next year!"

IT'S A FACT

You cannot start reversing cognitive decline yesterday; begin today.

Take your symptoms as a warning! Do something today! Without taking action, doing something different, or changing your habits, the symptoms next year will only be worse. It's always that way.

I've been practicing medicine for decades, and the only time symptoms change for the better is when we do something that causes it to happen. The natural progression of health is always downward. What is unknown is the rate of descent.

Common terms such as *mild cognitive impairment*, *age-associated memory impairment*, and *normal aging* are often thrown around when someone notices the symptoms. Those are warning bells that must be listened to. The time is always now to take action. The symptoms are usually reversible if you act soon enough. That's how you win at this game.

Tests You Can Take

Of the many tests you can take to confirm memory loss, one of my favorites is the MoCA (Montreal Cognitive Assessment test at www.mocatest.org). It's free to patients and available through an app, and it usually only takes about ten minutes to complete the thirty-question test. It's designed to help detect cognitive impairment and thus provide faster diagnosis.[3]

You can take many other tests, such as the MMSE (Mini Mental State Exam at www2.gov.bc.ca/assets/gov/health/practitioner-pro/bc-guidelines/cogimp-smmse.pdf) or the SAGE (Self-Administered Gerocognitive Exam). Some online memory assessment tests need an administrator, while others you can do completely by yourself.

For brain scans, the positron emission tomography (PET) scan is the best. You are given a radioactive form of glucose (sugar) called fluorodeoxyglucose (FDG) that is traced through your brain to show if you have reduced glucose metabolized in the hippocampus regions of your brain. A hallmark of Alzheimer's disease is a reduction in glucose metabolism in the brain, especially in the hippocampus region. The PET scan shows if that's happening; it can occur long before a diagnosis is made.

I often tell people experiencing significant memory loss to get a PET scan of the brain. The PET scan shows a consistent pattern with decreased activity in the temporal and parietal regions of the brain, even in the early stages of Alzheimer's disease. The hippocampus is a seahorse-shaped structure located in the brain's temporal lobe. A healthy hippocampus stores information temporarily in short-term memory. When the brain converts temporary memory to permanent memory, the hippocampus interacts with the cerebral cortex to encode the information into long-term storage. The PET scan can detect very mild changes that occur during early Alzheimer's disease.

Not long ago I sent one of my patients, a forty-five-year-old woman who was experiencing significant memory loss, to get a PET scan of her brain. The PET scan diagnosed her and helped her see what was going on in her brain. She immediately addressed her memory loss issues, and her PET scan twelve months later showed marked improvement.

The PET scan is 85 percent accurate in showing a reduction in glucose metabolism that signifies a brain struggling for fuel (glucose), which is always present in those with Alzheimer's at any level.[4] An amyloid PET scan measures the amount of amyloid beta protein deposition in the brain.

Believe it or not, you can also take a retinal imaging test. It makes sense since the retina is an extension of the brain, and these tests are much cheaper than a PET scan or amyloid PET scan. They can identify the amyloid plaque buildup in the retina, and you can identify the number of amyloid plaques and map their locations. Then, one year later, after a change in diet and lifestyle that optimizes nutrients and hormones, get rechecked to see if the number of plaques decreased. It's as simple as finding an ophthalmologist who offers retinal scanning.

Cerebral spinal fluid can also diagnose Alzheimer's, but not many patients choose that option.

Blood tests and urine tests do not show if you have Alzheimer's or dementia, but doctors request them to see if there are other conditions present (i.e., thyroid and other hormonal deficiencies or vitamin deficiencies) that might be causing or contributing to the symptoms. Doctors may also order other tests that measure inflammation, such as hs-CRP (high-sensitivity C-reactive protein).

I use blood and urine tests not only to check for other possible memory loss–causing factors but also to create a baseline for the patient. What nutrient and hormone levels are suboptimal? Are they insulin resistant? Is inflammation excessive? Do they have a toxic burden of heavy metals? Once I know these factors and more, we can create a plan. Knowing this information is beneficial because most people need to walk back, reverse, and undo their current diet and lifestyle.

I usually have patients get blood tests every three to six months at first, and then every six months to a year after things settle down. See appendix A for the list of tests and the target values for each test.

Depending on a person's need and budget, I usually tell patients who are testing for memory loss to start with online memory tests, such as the MoCA, then move up to retinal or PET scans. Most importantly, if you are taking tests to confirm what you already know, then it's past time that you take action to work on removing whatever is causing your memory loss.

Remember, if you think you already have memory problems, then do something about it. Being proactive is always the right move when dealing with the brain.

CHAPTER 4

WHAT CAN YOU DO ABOUT IT?

WITH ALZHEIMER'S, OR with any memory-related disease, for that matter, it's easy to feel hopeless and helpless when you read things such as, "No one knows exactly what causes Alzheimer's disease," or, "There's no known cure."[1] But you can do a lot about Alzheimer's and dementia. You can usually stop these deadly diseases in their tracks if you start early enough.

That's what we must do. Globally, if we don't take action, we will more than likely experience one of the greatest self-induced catastrophes known to man. Within thirty years the number of people in the United States living with Alzheimer's is expected to nearly triple.[2]

I think that number is too conservative, based on the current health trends and patients I see every day, but whether it's three times or ten times worse than today, it's already out of hand. According to the National Institute on Aging, the number of people with Alzheimer's doubles every five years past age sixty-five.[3]

IT'S A FACT

The "normal aging" of memory affects 40 percent of people in their fifties, 50 percent of people in their sixties, and 70 percent of people aged seventy and over.[4]

Unfortunately we aren't the best at reading warnings or taking preventive measures. For example, we all know obesity is bad for our health (it leads to more than thirty major diseases), but despite all that is known, repeated, marketed, and explained, the rates of obesity only keep climbing every single year.

That's the norm. People simply don't want to change their habits.

This means that it comes down to you. It's your choice. You live your life how you want to live it.

You Can Fight Against Alzheimer's and Dementia

In a nutshell, the best way to fight back against a sickness or disease is to remove whatever is causing it. Once you remove the source—whatever is causing the problems—the downward slide is usually slowed or stopped.

You fixed the problem!

Naturally, you replace what was bad with what is good, and the scales tip the other way. Your health improves, symptoms go away, and you usually recover.

It is said that virtually everyone with cognitive decline has at least one of these factors: insulin resistance, toxins, low oxygen levels, leaky gut, gum disease, chronic infections, deficiency in vitamin B12 or vitamin D, and heart disease.[5]

Those with hypertension, high cholesterol, and diabetes have an increased risk of dementia.[6] Smoking alone doubles your risk of Alzheimer's.[7]

Regardless of Alzheimer's or dementia, when you address any of those issues (i.e., insulin resistance, toxins, leaky gut, high cholesterol, and more), your health naturally improves. With Alzheimer's and dementia symptoms, it usually takes a few months to see improvement, but improvement happens! Sometimes it's even quicker for my patients, but six months is average.

Alzheimer's expert Dr. Dale Bredesen takes the position that Alzheimer's is a protective response against a bad environment. When the environment is good, there is no Alzheimer's.[8]

That is how you fight back! When you fix the environment, everything can change.

Again, Alzheimer's and dementia are not diseases you catch; they are your body's responses to what you are doing to it. Change what you are doing to your body, and your memory should improve.

You Can Turn Off the Alzheimer's Switch

Research has found that Alzheimer's has an amyloid precursor protein (APP) that acts as a switch that turns it on and thereby off. That's right! If you can turn it on, you can turn it off.

As it relates to your environment and fighting back against Alzheimer's and dementia, Dr. Bredesen found that if the environment in your body and brain is good (favorable), the Alzheimer's APP switch is off. That means your body usually has

- optimal levels of nutrients, hormones, and brain growth factors;
- minimal or no pathogens or inflammation;
- no insulin resistance;
- not been exposed to excessive toxins, dementogens, or heavy metals, and has a low toxic burden; and
- a normal homocysteine level (7 or lower).

But if the environment in your body and brain is bad (unfavorable), the switch is on. That means your body usually has

- low or inadequate nutrients, hormones, or brain growth factors;
- pathogens or inflammation present;
- insulin resistance present;
- exposure to excessive toxins, dementogens, or heavy metals; and
- homocysteine levels usually elevated.

Technically speaking, this switch is an individual protein (APP) that sticks out of each brain cell like the hair on your head. This protein will be cut with molecular "scissors" (called proteases) in different places, depending on your body and brain's environment.

If the APP protein is snipped off at a single spot (due to a good environment), the result is two peptides. Then your brain will grow, produce, and cause the growth of more synapses and neurons. Your brain loves it, and it is needed for good memory and cognition.

IT'S A FACT

Despite the billions of dollars spent, there is no known cure for Alzheimer's and dementia.

However, if the environment is unfavorable, the protein will be snipped in three different (all wrong) places, resulting in cellular death, cellular debris, downsizing, removing synapses, brain shrinkage, and amyloid buildup—all of which are directly associated with Alzheimer's disease.[9]

The norm these days is about 5 percent of people have Alzheimer's by age sixty-five, and it steadily increases to almost 50 percent by age eighty-five.[10] Who wants to be part of the norm? I for one do not!

The environment controls the switch, and you control the environment. Clearly, then, you are the one in control of the switch. Will you let it turn on, as most of the world is doing, or will you take the necessary steps to turn it off and keep it off?

It's up to you. The environment you create in and around your body and brain will be your answer.

You Can Stay Ahead of the Curve

Never letting the Alzheimer's switch turn on is the best answer. For most over fifty, the switch has already turned on, but you can turn it back off. If you are fifty years of age or older, most likely your hormones are suboptimal, low normal, or low, and that can flip the switch to start the brain downsizing.

However, regardless of your age, that switch can usually be turned off.

Looking back at the different types of Alzheimer's and dementia, it is evident that there are commonalities among them. There are usually four key underlying causes of a bad environment, which help flip the Alzheimer's switch.

The four factors are

1. chronic inflammation,
2. suboptimal levels of nutrients and hormones and brain growth factors,

3. toxins, and
4. insulin resistance.

Obviously, much can be said about these. Entire books can be written on each subject, and I've done it. But the point here is that when you deal with these four, you usually effectively stop or slow the advancement of Alzheimer's and dementia. That is how you stay ahead of the curve.

Of these four, chronic inflammation is probably the worst. It is at the root of most chronic diseases—not just Alzheimer's but also high blood pressure, autoimmune diseases, diabetes, asthma, rheumatoid arthritis, sinusitis, inflammatory bowel disease, chronic peptic ulcers, and cancers. These diseases are terrible, but it is especially bad that chronic inflammation causes your body to produce amyloid plaque, which builds up in your brain's hippocampus (near your temples).

If you have ongoing, chronic inflammation anywhere in your body, then you can expect amyloid production to build up in your brain, which will eventually lead to Alzheimer's disease. Quite simply, you need to lower inflammation, and lower it quickly!

Remember, it's all about your environment. When you have a healthy, thriving environment, the switch for Alzheimer's is usually turned off. Your brain cells are growing, synapses are being produced, your brain isn't shrinking, and your memory usually improves.

A nonhealthy environment, like a bad economy, negatively affects everything. In the brain, the cells downsize and degenerate, and synapses quit forming and degenerate, and the brain shrinks (atrophies). Memory problems increase as amyloid plaques and neurofibrillary tangles accumulate and damage and destroy brain cells and synapses.

IT'S A FACT

Having diabetes quadruples the risk of heart disease and strokes, and it increases the risk of Alzheimer's and dementia.[11]

Now that you know the four key factors that flip on the Alzheimer's switch, it only makes sense that improving your levels of nutrients, hormones, and brain growth factors; getting rid of toxins; and correcting insulin resistance are a vital part of keeping the Alzheimer's switch in the "off" position.

One amazing thing about the brain is that efforts to prevent cognitive decline also work to reverse existing cognitive decline. That is because the brain is always firing, ready to grow, and ready to heal. That's the way God made it, along with its five hundred trillion–plus synapses! These synapses are constantly communicating, which (if you ever wondered) is why the brain is only 2 percent of your total body mass yet uses 20 percent of your body's total energy supply.

Prevention can help reverse damage that's already done, which leads you to a long-term healthy, happy brain.

In the pages to come, you will learn more precisely how to prevent, slow, manage, stop, or reverse Alzheimer's and dementia if addressed soon enough.

CHAPTER 5

IS IT GENETIC?

YES, GENETIC FACTORS play a part in Alzheimer's and dementia. But even if your genes happen to be against you, there is still much you can do to prevent and reverse the disease, if addressed soon enough.

The specific memory gene that we are talking about is the ApoE4 gene. The ApoE4 gene gives instructions for making a protein called apolipoprotein E4. This protein then joins with fats to form lipoproteins. The lipoproteins then package cholesterol and other fats and transport them through the blood. If you have the ApoE4 gene, you are at the greatest risk for Alzheimer's and dementia, as well as heart attack and stroke.

An ApoE gene test at a lab (with your doctor's order for it) will give you your results. I request this all the time for my patients. It is the strongest known genetic risk factor for Alzheimer's disease. You can't remove the gene from your body, but you can do *a lot* to prevent Alzheimer's and dementia even if you have the gene.

ApoE4: One Lump or Two?

Odds are you don't have either one or two copies of the ApoE4 gene. You see, each of us has two ApoE genes, and we get one from each parent. And since there are three main ApoE types (ApoE2, ApoE3, and ApoE4), there are six possible combinations.

These variations have been studied, and we know what the odds are.

- ApoE2/ApoE2: 1 percent of the population
- ApoE2/ApoE3: 10 percent of the population
- ApoE3/ApoE3: 64 percent of the population
- ApoE2/ApoE4: 2 percent of the population

- ApoE3/ApoE4: 18 percent of the population
- ApoE4/ApoE4: 5 percent of the population[1]

All combined, you can see that about 20 percent of the population carries one ApoE4 gene, and only 5 percent carries two copies of the ApoE4 gene. I've seen the percentage of people who have two copies of the ApoE4 gene reported as just 2–3 percent, but whether it's 2 percent or 5 percent, it's a small number who have two copies of the ApoE4 gene.

Despite all the research and the scare factor of knowing you might or do carry one or two copies of the ApoE4 gene, know this: *the ApoE4 gene does not guarantee that you will even get Alzheimer's or dementia.*

The ApoE4 gene causes a reduction in glucose metabolism in the brain (sluggish brain metabolism), which may eventually create much greater inflammation within the brain. The ApoE gene also produces a protein that transports fats and cholesterol throughout the body, creates cell membranes, moves molecules within the cell, and generates energy.[2]

IT'S A FACT

To prevent Alzheimer's disease, you must know your ApoE gene status.

However, your brain is designed by God for speed. Did you know that about a wine bottle's worth of blood is pumped through your brain every sixty seconds?[3] That's a lot of pumping, and it's moving quickly through the trillions of synapses in your brain.

But if your brain's metabolism is slowed down, your brain eventually pays the price. You begin to have decreased fuel, energy, and nutrients, which leads to increased inflammation in the brain. You eventually flip on the Alzheimer's switch, and your brain starts to downsize, sacrificing neurons and synapses, accumulating amyloid plaques and neurofibrillary tangles as it downsizes.

As you already know, prolonged inflammation is terrible for your body. For the brain, when inflammation is excessive, those plaques and tangles form, and brain cells begin to die. This is where the ApoE4 gene shows its direct impact. Consider these statistics for the US population and their risk of getting Alzheimer's:

- Those with no ApoE4 gene have a 9 percent risk.
- Those with one ApoE4 gene have about a 30 percent risk.
- Those with two copies of the ApoE4 gene have more than a 50 percent risk.[4]

How does that translate into age for someone who develops Alzheimer's or dementia?

- Those with no ApoE4 gene won't typically see symptoms until their late sixties or seventies.
- Those with one ApoE4 gene typically begin to show signs of Alzheimer's in their late fifties or sixties.[5]

What about someone with two copies of the ApoE4 gene? It can be much earlier. I've had patients in their early forties who came in with memory-related issues, only to discover after getting their blood tested that they had two copies of the ApoE4 gene.

They may not have noticed it earlier, but the brain was already paying the price. Autopsies of young people (ages twenty-two to forty-six) with the ApoE4 gene showed a 36 percent increase in plaques and tangles compared with those without the ApoE4 gene.[6]

Thankfully, at my patients' young age and because it was caught early, they could do a lot of work to repair and prevent further damage, and their prospects looked great afterward. Most patients who start early enough can usually protect the brain from Alzheimer's if the issues are caught and corrected early enough. It's amazing!

IT'S A FACT

About 33 percent of what determines successful aging is genes; the rest is your environment, especially the foods and lifestyle you choose.[7]

But since so few people have checked their ApoE gene, most ApoE4 carriers don't even know they have it. This means they are not taking preventive measures at the most important time—when they could and should be doing something about it!

Personally, my ApoE gene score is ApoE3/ApoE4. (My wife, Mary, is ApoE3/ApoE3.) I received the one ApoE4 gene from my father's side of the family. That means statistically, I'm in the 30 percent risk category, but that also means I am (and have been for many years) taking many preventive measures to keep that APP switch from flipping to Alzheimer's disease.

Everything you read in this book, I'm already doing. From diet to sleep, exercise to lifestyle, less stress to balanced hormones, and avoiding toxins to taking supplements and brain supplements, I'm doing it. I fully intend to live a long, productive life.

So can you.

Mixing ApoE4 With Head Trauma

The ApoE gene has an inconvenient way of working itself into many aspects of our lives. It may even limit your choices of sports and professions, both for you and your family.

I suggest that people with the ApoE4 gene avoid contact sports such as football, boxing, rugby, mixed martial arts, kickboxing, even soccer, and careers such as race car driving, movie stunting, or motorbike racing.

Why? Because when you have head trauma, your body produces the same amyloid plaques that Alzheimer's patients have. And if you have the ApoE4 gene and have head trauma, it's even worse!

Moderate head injury (with loss of consciousness or post-traumatic amnesia for more than thirty minutes but less than twenty-four hours) has been found to double the risk of developing Alzheimer's. But when that person has the ApoE4 gene, the risk of developing Alzheimer's multiplies tenfold![8]

That is because the plaques and tangles that build up after head trauma, along with the ApoE4 gene associated with sluggish brain metabolism and more inflammation, cause even greater damage than usual. At ten times the usual damage, that is a lot!

If you have someone in the family with Alzheimer's and your kids want to play contact sports, you should have the ApoE gene test to check for the ApoE4 gene. (See appendix A.) You can check for the gene at any age, but if both parents are tested and don't carry the ApoE4 gene, you know the child does not either.

It's not a matter of being weak or walking in fear; it's simply that the ApoE4 gene can harm our brains in ways we cannot control. The best move is to get tested, then move on from there.

Mixing ApoE4 With High Cholesterol

Another way that the ApoE4 gene harms our bodies has to do with our cholesterol. The ApoE4 gene causes our cells to excessively absorb dietary fat, elevating cholesterol levels.[9] Limiting the bad fats (excessive saturated fats, trans fats, and others) and increasing the good fats (olive oil, avocado oil, nuts, seeds, fish, and others) is the best move.

The ApoE protein carries cholesterol in the blood, so when there are high blood cholesterol levels, the ApoE gene moves it around even more, increasing your risk of heart disease and stroke.[10] Instead of letting the body remove the cholesterol, the ApoE4 gene keeps it in circulation and increases your level of LDL cholesterol, which is atherogenic cholesterol.

If you are wondering if statin drugs that lower cholesterol will lower Alzheimer's risk as well, you are correct. Statin drugs that lower cholesterol have been found to help decrease the risk of Alzheimer's by as much as 70 percent.[11] However, our brains also need cholesterol. If statins lower your cholesterol levels too much, it can harm your brain in new ways.

I've had many patients who feel as if they are in a constant daze with brain fog. They struggle mentally and can't focus, think clearly, or make decisions. For them, it wasn't a memory-loss issue. Rather, they were taking a dose of statin that was too high and was lowering their cholesterol too much. We lowered their statin intake until their cholesterol level got above 150 (between 150 and 200 is the best range), and they became mentally sharp again and the brain fog left.

IT'S A FACT

"Dr. Richard Mayeux and research associates at Columbia University found that people who have blacked out for an hour or more following a head trauma have a twofold increased risk of developing Alzheimer's disease down the road. If such a person also has the APOE-4 genetic risk for Alzheimer's disease, their overall risk for the disease increases to tenfold."[12]

For example, if a patient is on the statin drug Crestor at 40 milligrams, I may lower them in 10-milligram increments until their cholesterol level rises just above 150. I know they want to lower their cholesterol, and many push it below 100, but that is usually too low to maintain a good memory. A cholesterol level below 150 is in and of itself associated with memory decline, so don't do that. The brain must have sufficient cholesterol to function properly.

If you have the ApoE4 gene, you need to lower your cholesterol levels to around 150.

IT'S A FACT

Smokers beware: if you smoke and have the ApoE4 gene, you are at additional risk for heart disease.[13]

Mixing ApoE4 With Sugar

As you know, foods high in sugar and high in carbohydrates (such as desserts, cereals, syrups, breads, white rice, pasta, ice cream, candy, and many other foods) cause insulin levels to spike.

And since correcting insulin resistance is vital to keeping the

Alzheimer's switch in the "off" position, it means that high-sugar and high-carb foods must be eliminated from your diet, especially if you have the ApoE4 gene.

Someone with the ApoE4 gene is genetically predisposed to suffering from insulin resistance at an earlier age (as early as their teens!). The ApoE4 gene makes things exponentially worse. Patients with the ApoE4 gene usually have a decrease in the metabolism of glucose in the brain, especially in the temporal areas, where Alzheimer's affects the brain, in their thirties.[14] The answer is to eat foods that don't spike your insulin levels, as with a healthy keto or Mediterranean diet (discussed in greater detail in chapter 25). The ApoE4 gene does not mix well with sugar or carbs.

Mixing ApoE4 With Alcohol

Heavy drinking is known to increase many different health risks, including Alzheimer's and dementia, but there is something else that everyone with the ApoE4 gene must know: any amount of alcohol increases the risk of Alzheimer's and dementia for those with the ApoE4 gene.[15] Heavy, moderate, or light drinking is bad. Simply put, alcohol and the ApoE4 gene should not mix.

Though red wine is often recommended for its health benefits, I would certainly not recommend it if you carry two copies of the ApoE4 gene, and then only sparingly (if at all) if you carry one copy of the ApoE4 gene.

By *sparingly*, I mean one small glass of dry red wine once or twice a week. Yes, red wine with dinner (one to two glasses for men and less for women) is commonly recommended as a healthy option,[16] but for ApoE4 carriers, with the increased health risks, I don't think it's healthy or recommendable.

We talk more about alcohol and the ApoE4 gene in chapter 11.

IT'S A FACT

It is estimated that 36 percent of people age eighty-five and older are affected by Alzheimer's disease.[17]

If You Have the ApoE4 Gene

Most doctors see their patients for ten to fifteen minutes and then after a brief consult tell them to come back next year. And if they prescribe a drug to help with memory, that does nothing to stop the progression of Alzheimer's or dementia.

Brain expert Dr. Gary Small found that everyone with the ApoE4 gene showed a decline in brain function with each subsequent PET scan of the brain's parietal and temporal memory areas.[18] Every PET scan showed that things were getting worse—every single one!

Because patients with the ApoE4 gene are at such a high risk of Alzheimer's and dementia, I can't say enough how important it is to follow the Healthy Brain Zone protocol that this book outlines. Doing so will reduce inflammation, lower cholesterol, heal leaky gut, correct insulin resistance, correct key nutritional deficiencies, optimize nutrient levels, optimize hormone levels, and treat chronic infections.

It will also help you establish regular exercise; practice intermittent fasting; follow a ketogenic, low-carb diet with lots of green veggies and fiber; detoxify; learn to cope with stress; and get refreshing, well-oxygenated sleep.

With the ApoE4 gene, prevention is the best thing to do, and the time to start is now.

PART II:
THE TOP TEN DEMENTOGENS THAT HURT YOUR BRAIN

If Alzheimer's and dementia are the result of the environment we create, sustain, or provide our bodies, then it follows that we can identify what within the environment is causing the body to react—and reverse it! And that is exactly what we are doing. When you fix the environment, the symptoms usually go away.

These ten key dementogens are known causes of Alzheimer's and dementia. A dementogen is a chemical, heavy metal, toxin, or substance that causes dementia. There are many other dementogens, but I believe these are the most important ones to address. World-renowned brain expert Dale Bredesen says there are thirty-six causes of Alzheimer's and dementia. I believe we will find even more in time, but however many there are, the goal is always the same: to remove these dementogens from our lives. Why? Doing so has been found to many times stop these diseases in their tracks.

CHAPTER 6

DEMENTOGEN 1: HEAVY METALS

HEAVY METALS ARE a dementogen (dementia-causing agent) that comes in many different forms. Of course, nobody goes around eating, drinking, or exposing themselves to these heavy metals on purpose. Nonetheless, these metals may eventually get into our bodies and cause untold damage.

There are two problems with heavy metals: (1) they are toxic and cause disease, including Alzheimer's and dementia, and (2) they accumulate over time. As they build up, our bodies store these toxins in the worst places—our brains, blood, bones, and fat.[1] They slowly saturate the cell membrane and prevent the body from doing its job.[2]

Humans aren't the only ones accumulating heavy metals. Plants and animals do so as well. And if those plants and animals are part of the food chain, then our bodies must deal with them even more so.

Over time, the slowly accumulated toxins begin to have their disease-causing effect. Because it happens so slowly, the results are unexpected and may appear "suddenly." Had preventive measures been taken, the toxins never would have accumulated and the subsequent diseases would not have gained a foothold. Prevention is truly the best cure!

IT'S A FACT

Studies have failed to confirm that exposure to aluminum through such things as antiperspirants, pans, cans, and antacids causes Alzheimer's disease.[3]

Here are the most common heavy metals known to cause, among many other things, Alzheimer's and dementia.

Heavy Metal 1: Mercury

Of all the heavy metals, mercury is the worst. It has been known to cause countless health problems, including the plaques and tangles in the brain always found in Alzheimer's patients.[4]

Our primary sources of mercury are the silver fillings in our teeth and fish, but mercury is also in drinking water, air, oceans, and soil, as well as in certain vaccinations and cosmetics. Some occupations, such as mining, have higher levels of mercury exposure than average.

IT'S A FACT

Mercury, lead, cadmium, and arsenic can be found in tap water, and drinking tap water containing these heavy metals "is becoming a major health concern for public and health care professionals."[5] Reverse osmosis is an effective way to remove heavy metals from water.[6]

Mercury in silver fillings

In 2007, the World Health Organization (WHO) stated that our biggest daily exposure to mercury is from our silver fillings (dental amalgams).[7] And dentists still use it to this day! About 55 percent of the silver fillings in our teeth are mercury, and each filling releases one microgram of mercury per day into the body.[8] If you have five or ten fillings, that adds up! The answer is to get the fillings replaced with non-mercury fillings. I suggest doing only one or two at a time, not all at once, and finding a mercury-free dentist, such as one from the International Academy of Oral Medicine and Toxicology (IAOMT). One study found that after twenty years, your average amalgam "silver" filling can lose up to 95 percent of its mercury content.[9] Where does this mercury go? It accumulates in fatty organs, including the brain. Older silver fillings may be less toxic than earlier thought.

IT'S A FACT

What is a half-life? In terms of health, half-life describes how long it takes 50 percent of a substance to be cleared from your body.

Mercury in fish

If you eat a lot of fish, you may be at an increased risk of mercury exposure. Big fish have the most mercury because they live longer and accumulate more in their flesh over time. Also, these mercury levels are rising. For example, the mercury in tuna has been rising by 4 percent every year.[10] High-mercury fish include shark, swordfish, marlin, orange roughy, king mackerel, tilefish, and bigeye tuna. Smaller fish and seafood are best to eat, as they are lower on the food chain and have collected less mercury than bigger fish. One common, quick way to choose healthy fish is the acronym SMASH, which stands for salmon, mackerel, anchovies, sardines, and herring. But black sea bass, tongol tuna, catfish, shrimp, clams, flounder, tilapia, cod, crab, trout, oysters, scallops, squid, and whitefish (among many others) are also low in mercury. Wild (not farm-raised) is always best.

Mercury in cosmetics

Some soaps, lotions, and creams contain mercury. Look at the label (if there is no label, that is suspect as well) for the words *mercurous chloride*, *calomel*, *mercuric*, *mercurio*, or *mercury*.[11] If those words are present, so is mercury. Find another product.

Mercury penetrates the blood-brain barrier (which separates the brain from blood) and causes damage.[12] When the blood-brain barrier is damaged, toxins enter the brain more easily, and it only worsens from there (just like a leaky gut).

The half-life of mercury in the brain lasts from a few years to several decades.[13] That is a long time, which means a lot of exposure and damage.

If you are wondering if it's possible to remove the mercury that has built up in the brain, the answer is yes! It's not like mercury and other heavy metals settle at the bottom of the brain or other organs, but a process called chelation can remove heavy metals from your body.

Chelation uses chemically inert, nontoxic agents to bond with the metal ions, and then both are secreted out of the body. These agents can be given by mouth, with an IV, via injection, or rectally.

The IV method is usually the most effective and thus most common. When the special chelation agents enter your bloodstream, they bind with the heavy metals in your brain and elsewhere in your body to form a new chemical, which is then taken to your kidneys and passed through your urine.

For most people, I suggest focusing first on reducing their exposure to mercury, as that will make the biggest impact. But for those who show symptoms of mercury toxicity or have blood work that shows high levels of mercury, consider finding a doctor who is experienced in using dimercaptosuccinic acid (DMSA) or dimercaptopropane sulfonate (DMPS) chelation agents or other effective chelators of mercury, such as glutathione and alpha-lipoic acid.

Not everyone needs to do chelation, but it is a necessary step for some.

IT'S A FACT

Symptoms of mercury toxicity:

» *physical tremors*

» *memory and concentration problems*

» *muscle weakness*

» *metallic taste in the mouth*

» *feeling uncoordinated*

» *changes in vision, hearing, and speech*

» *difficulty walking or standing*

» *depression, nervousness, or anxiety*

» *numbness*

» *irritability or mood changes*[14]

Heavy Metal 2: Arsenic

Over time, the accumulation of arsenic in your body can affect every organ, including your brain, and has been found to lead to cancer, kidney and liver disease, numbness of limbs, hearing issues, gut problems, and much more.[15] It also causes an increase in the plaques and tangles that are so closely associated with Alzheimer's disease.[16]

Arsenic is in groundwater and soil, which means it can reach everywhere. Unfortunately arsenic is both odorless and tasteless. Because arsenic is often found in groundwater, it's also found in drinking water and the many foods that use that water.

That's why arsenic is often discovered in rice, chicken, dairy products, beef, pork, grains, apple juice, grape juice, wine, vegetables, and even baby formula and cereal bars (from brown rice syrup, which is used as a sweetener). If you eat a steady diet of these foods, you may have arsenic in your system.

Regarding the brain, arsenic reacts with brain cells, displacing certain elements and changing the cells' function,[17] and that's not a good thing at all! Arsenic is literally a poison to the hippocampus, the very area of your brain associated with short-term memory.[18]

IT'S A FACT

Arsenic in the United States is found primarily in the Western states, with some drinking water having arsenic levels far above the maximum allowed.[19]

Arsenic can be both organic and inorganic. Our bodies do not typically absorb the organic type (in fish and other seafood) at all, making it less of a health risk.[20] However, the inorganic type (in groundwater, foods, and more) is bad because our bodies cannot excrete it completely. Though inorganic arsenic has a short half-life of between four hours and four days, the long-term exposure and accumulated buildup really harm our bodies.

Arsenic is naturally occurring, but we also used it years ago as a pesticide to eliminate the boll weevil in the cotton fields. Many fields that used to grow cotton are now used to grow rice and other food crops. The arsenic is still present in the soil and will be present in the rice or other crops grown in the soil. This heavy metal has a way of staying put, which means it continues to affect us. Long-term exposure to drinking water with arsenic, even at low levels, has been associated with cognitive dysfunction.[21]

For recent or chronic exposure to arsenic, the twenty-four-hour urine collection for arsenic is a good test.

To get it out of your body, I always suggest first focusing on reducing exposure to arsenic, as that will make the biggest impact. But if you have symptoms of arsenic poisoning or have blood work that shows high levels of arsenic, use chelation agents: DMSA, DMPS, and penicillamine. Also, choose organic foods, including rice, chicken, and others.

IT'S A FACT

When the neurons in your brain age or die, your brain shrinks in size.[22]

HEAVY METAL 3: LEAD

Though mercury is ten times more toxic to your neurons than lead,[23] lead is itself a very dangerous heavy metal. Some even say it was the lowly lead water pipes that contributed to the decline and eventual downfall of the mighty Roman Empire!

We don't use lead pipes anymore, but we are still exposed to lead through drinking water, gasoline, paint, batteries, some canned foods, cigarette smoke, cosmetics (i.e., lipstick, eyeliner), some water pipes, and even children's toys.

Lead is also in the soil and old buildings. Lead-based paint has been banned for residential use since 1978, but it's still around. Think dust. Every big city in the world existed before 1978, which means that the dust in these cities still includes lead in the old paint particles. It's everywhere in big cities, and we breathe it every day.

Inhaled lead will work its way into the body, but most lead poisoning occurs through what we eat or drink. We absorb about 5–15 percent of the lead on its way through our digestive system; that lead then travels throughout our bodies and settles in our organs and bones.[24]

The half-life of lead is only about thirty-five days, but lead that settles in organs and bones can stick around for a couple of decades and even as long as fifty years![25] That is not good at all!

Also, when most women reach fifty years of age, their sex hormone levels drop, and many women start losing bone. Lead stored in their bones is then leached out of the bones as they develop osteopenia or osteoporosis.

Symptoms of lead poisoning for adults include

- abdominal, joint, and muscle pain;
- difficulty remembering or concentrating;
- headache;
- high blood pressure;
- miscarriage, stillbirth, or premature birth;
- mood disorders; and
- reduced sperm count and abnormal sperm.[26]

The symptoms are even worse for children. Specifically, regarding the brain, lead has been found to cause

- decreased learning,
- decreased memory,
- decreased verbal ability,
- impaired fine motor coordination,
- impaired hearing,
- impaired speech, and
- low IQ.[27]

As you might expect, the elderly population (ages fifty to seventy) suffers the most from long-term chronic exposure to lead.[28] Quite simply, lead exposure adds up as the lead settles in organs and bones over time.

IT'S A FACT

Recommended chelation therapy per heavy metal:

» *mercury: DMSA and DMPS*

» *arsenic: DMSA, DMPS, penicillamine*

» *lead: succimer, BAL, CaNa2EDTA*

» *cadmium: ethylenediaminetetraacetic acid (EDTA), DMPS, DMSA*[29]

This prolonged exposure to lead speeds up the rates of cognitive decline, the telltale plaque and tangles of Alzheimer's disease, and even increases the chances of Parkinson's disease.[30]

A simple blood test is the most common way to see if you have high amounts of lead in your body. At one time, anything above 10 mcg/dL (micrograms per deciliter) for adults and 5 mcg/dL for children was considered high.[31] The CDC has since said that lead levels in the blood of children should be less than 3.5 mcg/dL.[32] (See appendix A.)

To get it out of your body, I always suggest first focusing on reducing exposure to lead, as that will make the biggest impact, but if you have symptoms of lead poisoning or have blood work that shows high levels of lead, use chelation agents: succimer, British anti-Lewisite (BAL), and CaNa2EDTA.

Heavy Metal 4: Cadmium

Cadmium, though not as well known, is also toxic to our bodies. It is naturally occurring, but because it is water-soluble, cadmium can easily travel from soil to plants to you.[33]

Add that cadmium has a half-life of twenty to forty years, and it's easy to see how its accumulation (typically in the kidneys and liver) can lead to health issues, especially as we age.

This usually results in hypertension, kidney and bone issues, blood disorders, lung damage, a loss of smell, a higher cancer risk, and several neurological diseases.[34]

IT'S A FACT

Shellfish, kidney, liver, mushrooms, and root crops contain especially high levels of cadmium.[35]

More and more studies of the brain are finding that cadmium is closely associated with the accumulation of Alzheimer's plaques.[36]

The tobacco plant has higher levels of cadmium than most other plants, thus making cigarette smoking probably the number one source of cadmium exposure worldwide. Consequently, it's been found that smokers can have four to five times higher cadmium concentrations in their blood than nonsmokers.[37] If you or those you know need another reason to quit smoking, this could be it.

Cadmium may be naturally occurring, but we increase our exposure through paints that contain cadmium, chemical factories, the steel industry, zinc production, waste incineration, some fertilizer manufacturing, the handling of rechargeable batteries, and more.[38]

But that's not all. Cadmium is also in chocolate! It's in the cacao bean, but the higher the cacao level (the darker the chocolate), usually the lower the cadmium. Higher cacao levels of chocolate are healthier anyway, making the lower cadmium levels just another reason to enjoy darker chocolate (more than 75–85 percent).

High cadmium levels cause almost no symptoms (unless highly exposed via industrial exposure). With dangerous levels of cadmium, diseases such as heart attack, kidney failure, and osteoporosis can occur without much warning. Smokers who eat regular, conventionally grown foods are probably toxic with cadmium.[39]

Again, a simple blood or urine test will determine if you have excessive cadmium in your body. (See appendix A.)

To get it out of your body, I always suggest first focusing on reducing exposure to cadmium, as that will make the biggest impact, but if you have symptoms of cadmium poisoning or have blood work or urine tests that show high levels of cadmium, use chelation agents: EDTA, DMPS, or DMSA.

To find a doctor trained in chelation therapy to remove heavy metals, including mercury, arsenic, lead, and cadmium, go to acam.org. Follow directions and choose the specialty "Chelation Therapy." Make sure your practitioner is certified in chelation therapy.

Infrared sauna therapy also helps to mobilize mercury, arsenic, lead, and cadmium and remove them from the body. See chapter 18 for more information.

Glutathione is the "body's master detoxifier" and helps the body eliminate mercury, arsenic, lead, and cadmium. N-acetylcysteine, liposomal glutathione, or Cellgevity (see appendix F) are effective glutathione-boosting supplements. For more information on this, refer to my book *Toxic Relief.*

CHAPTER 7

DEMENTOGEN 2: ENVIRONMENTALLY ACQUIRED ILLNESSES

WHAT ARE ENVIRONMENTALLY acquired illnesses? This broad term is being used more and more to describe the diseases that cause chronic inflammation, all of which lead to an increased risk of Alzheimer's and dementia.

In particular, we are talking about chronic inflammation caused by mold, Lyme disease, Lyme disease coinfections, toxic chemicals, and heavy metals. Thankfully, getting sick from mold and Lyme disease is relatively uncommon. Technically, Lyme disease is an infection rather than an environmentally acquired illness, but it is often grouped as such.

Not only do the carriers of Lyme disease (primarily ticks that carry it from their infected hosts) bring Lyme disease, but they also carry such diseases as babesiosis, anaplasmosis, relapsing fever, Rocky Mountain spotted fever, bartonellosis, ehrlichiosis, and others. All these diseases are coinfections of Lyme disease. (Coinfection is acquiring multiple diseases from a single carrier.)

Dr. Neil Nathan, an expert on mold illness and treating patients with toxic inflammation, noted that about 80 percent of his sick patients who suffer from toxic inflammation have mold as the root cause and 20 percent have Lyme disease as the cause, and many have both.[1]

A weakened immune system leads to other infections, so by the time people see a doctor, they often suffer from a confusing jumble of diseases with a wide variety of symptoms. For those with chronic Lyme disease, most have one other disease, and 30 percent have two or more![2] As a result, it can take a while to diagnose and treat the chronic inflammation associated with these environmentally acquired illnesses, but if you have them, it's worth the effort!

With mold, it is important to note that an estimated five hundred thousand patients in the United States each year have Alzheimer's symptoms that are caused by molds.[3] Remove the mold and fix the chronic inflammation that the mold is causing, and the Alzheimer's symptoms usually go away. That is why getting to the root of the problem is the only correct way to deal with something causing any memory-related illness.

Lyme disease and Lyme disease coinfections can also produce symptoms that look a lot like Alzheimer's. Actor and musician Kris Kristofferson is a great example. He was diagnosed in his late sixties with fibromyalgia but was not checked for Lyme disease, though he no doubt had it. Things got worse, and eventually he was diagnosed with Alzheimer's.

This continued for three years, with treatments and drugs by two neurologists, until an MRI and a spinal tap ruled out Alzheimer's. He had Lyme disease all along, and treating his Lyme disease restored his memory!

Getting tested for Lyme disease or its possible coinfections may be a good move if you have been diagnosed with fibromyalgia or one of the coinfection diseases, or if you have memory loss and your doctor hasn't ruled out Lyme disease or Lyme disease coinfections.

Why Mold Can Be Toxic

The symptoms of mold toxicity are like none other. Only those who have had them can describe or empathize with someone else suffering from it. Symptoms of mold toxicity vary but include

- appetite swings,
- body temperature dysregulation,
- chest tightness and pain,
- cognitive impairment,
- depression with fatigue,
- disequilibrium,
- dizziness,
- electric shock sensations,
- excessive thirst,

- frequent urination,
- gastrointestinal symptoms (diarrhea, constipation, nausea, vomiting, bloating, gas, abdominal pain),
- headaches,
- ice pick–like pains (especially headaches),
- impotence,
- joint and muscle pain,
- a metallic taste in the mouth,
- mood swings,
- muscle weakness,
- night sweats,
- numbness,
- odd tics and spasms,
- seizure-like events,
- sensitivity to bright light,
- severe anxiety,
- skin sensitivity to touch,
- tingling in different parts of the body,
- vibrating or pulsing sensations that run up and down your spine, and
- weight gain.[4]

People with many of these symptoms are most likely diagnosed with fibromyalgia, chronic fatigue syndrome, or maybe even depression. But it's usually due to mold toxins!

Here is the interesting part: mold is toxic to about 25 percent of the world's population! It turns out that about 75 percent of us create an antibody that binds to the mold and gets rid of it. The remaining 25 percent of the population does not have the genetic ability to make this antibody and flush out the mold toxins.[5]

As with heavy metals, the mold toxins accumulate over time. These toxins dissolve into fat and water, moving through the body and brain to create nonstop inflammation.[6] It only gets progressively worse over time. The body is on constant alert with inflammation and cannot stop its own downward spiral because it can't expel the mold toxins.

This chronic inflammation makes mold (and Lyme disease and the Lyme disease coinfections) a dementogen because it all eventually leads to Alzheimer's and dementia. The brain ends up paying a terrible price.

Testing for Mold

How do you know if you are part of the 25 percent or 75 percent? Having the symptoms or not is one way of knowing. Another is to get your blood tested (at Labcorp, Quest Diagnostics, or another company) for several markers. I recommend Dr. Ritchie Shoemaker's website (survivingmold.com) and his protocol for dealing with mold. He even has a list of trained physicians who can help if you are part of that 25 percent.

According to Dr. Shoemaker, you want to look for the following markers and ranges in your blood work.

- HLA Genotyping (I include this in appendix A.)
- MSH—normal range: 35–81 pg/mL
- ADH—normal range: 1.0–13.3 pg/mL
- Osmolality—normal range: 280–300 mosmol
- TGF-beta-1—normal range: less than 2380 pg/mL
- C4a—normal range: 0–2830 ng/mL
- MMP-9—normal range: 85–332 ng/mL[7]

I commonly request this blood work for mold patients.

As for testing your home for mold, even the Bible had a protocol for mold. If you haven't read the last half of Leviticus 14 (vv. 33–57) in a while, it's an interesting read, especially from the perspective of how accurate and effective such a treatment plan would have been back then and even today.

Today there are many different options if you think you may need to test your home for mold. You can do tests yourself, send in samples, or have professionals come out and do the tests. Besides seeing mold or smelling a musty smell, what you are testing is the dust in your house. If it's present, mold will usually be in the dust, and the samples taken from various places in the house will confirm it.

One option I often recommend is the Environmental Relative Moldiness Index (ERMI) lab service, but many services can help test your home for mold toxins.

Treatment Options for Mold

Several years ago I had a mother (about age thirty-five) of two school-age children (around ages seven and nine) come in with a strange set of symptoms. Most of all, she complained of splitting headaches (as with an ice pick) and feeling as if her brain were turned off. She could hardly function, her children needed her, and the headaches would shut her down.

Chronic inflammation was undoubtedly part of the problem, as that is what mold causes for 25 percent of the population who don't have the genetic ability to self-bind the toxins and pass them out of the body. She also suffered from irritable bowel syndrome (IBS) from all the mold toxins in her gut. I checked the lab tests on Dr. Shoemaker's list, and most of hers were out of range, indicating mold toxins. We started a process to bind and remove the mold toxins from her gut using the binder cholestyramine. I also put her on a special antibiotic nose spray (BEG nasal spray) to help deal with persistent sinus issues caused by multiple antibiotic resistant coagulase negative staphylococci (MARCoNS).

Her husband wasn't affected at all, but she was. He was part of the 75 percent that had the genes that could handle mold, and she was part of the 25 percent that could not.

While this was happening, they also ordered an ERMI test. Mold experts came out and took dust samples from various rooms. The score proved that they had mold throughout their home.

IT'S A FACT

Molds make toxins called mycotoxins, which enter your body through your lungs, skin, or gut (from foods you eat). Usually you inhale the mycotoxins.[8]

A few years earlier there had been some water damage from a broken pipe. The water damage had not been properly remediated, and mold and mold toxins were present in the drywall.

They all moved to a hotel for a few weeks while the house was properly remediated for mold.

In addition to the doctor visits, medications, and careful mold removal in the home, she also set up special air filters, which remove mold toxins and other contaminants in her bedroom and living room. She spent most of her time at home in these two rooms.

Within a few weeks her headaches were gone! Then, over a few months, her brain turned back on, her memory was restored, and her IBS cleared up. She was a changed woman.

About a year went by, and then she called my offices. Both of her children were beginning to have the same symptoms. They were obviously (from her genes) part of the 25 percent, but with the mom having no symptoms and the house cleaned and the air filter in place, it didn't make sense.

It was their school. There was mold in the school walls from previous water damage that had not been remediated well enough. Same issue, just a different location. (Office buildings can do the same for those who are part of the 25 percent.)

I have seen people walk inside a building and start feeling sick within five to ten minutes. That's how sensitive they are. So imagine how sick they can become if they live there, go to school there, or work there.

The answer for her children? They transferred to another school, and within a few months the symptoms were gone.

For adults, changing jobs, working from home, or moving is at times the only way to escape the never-ending cycle of exposure to mold toxins.

Not addressing the issue will never fix it. Symptoms will usually get worse and worse, and eventually it will damage the brain. (Lyme disease and Lyme disease coinfections will do the same thing.) I recommend IGeneX lab tests for Lyme and coinfections.

Someone who is properly trained needs to handle the treatment for mold, Lyme disease, and Lyme disease coinfections. Doctors trained by Dr. Shoemaker (survivingmold.com) can be one such option.

Whatever the "environmentally acquired illness" might be, in the end there is hope!

CHAPTER 8

DEMENTOGEN 3: ANTICHOLINERGIC MEDICATIONS

CONTINUED USE OF certain medications can increase the risk of Alzheimer's and dementia. Most people taking these drugs are age sixty-five and older and taking the medications for far longer than they should.

The usual ailments they are trying to treat include

- allergies,
- depression,
- dizziness,
- epilepsy,
- GI disorders,
- glaucoma,
- insomnia,
- irritable bowel syndrome (IBS),
- mucus secretion,
- muscle relaxation,
- nausea/seasickness,
- Parkinson's disease,
- schizophrenia,
- spastic bladder, and
- urinary incontinence.

Usually people with these issues begin to take medications and keep taking the medications for years and years. The short-term fix becomes a long-term treatment plan—but these medications are not meant for that.

Seldom would I recommend using anticholinergic or certain antihistamine medications, such as Benadryl, for longer than three months and virtually never longer than six months. Claritin, Zyrtec, and Allegra are antihistamines but are not anticholinergic. Anticholinergic medications block the neurotransmitter acetylcholine, which is involved in learning and memory. Ideally, during that time, we are supposed to find answers, such as finding a natural alternative, using a different medication that's not an anticholinergic medication, eating differently, revising bad habits, beginning an exercise program, and the like. No bandage solution is ever meant to be permanent.

IT'S A FACT

Anticholinergic medications may increase the risk of dementia by more than 50 percent, and 20–50 percent of Americans age sixty-five and older take at least one anticholinergic medication.[1]

I know people who have continued using anticholinergic medications for five to ten years, even longer! Those over age sixty-five who use these medications for more than three years have a 54 percent increased risk of Alzheimer's and dementia.[2] Prolonged use is bad for the brain.

Here is a list of just some of the medications with moderate to high anticholinergic activity that can impair your memory and predispose you to Alzheimer's and dementia over time.

Category	Brand Name	Generic Name
Analgesic	Demerol Ultram	meperidine tramadol
Antihistamine	Benadryl Atarax Chlortripolon	diphenhydramine hydroxyzine chlorpheniramine
Incontinence	Ditropan Detrol LA	oxybutynin tolterodine
Antiparkinson	Cogentin Symmetrel	benztropine amantadine
Antipsychotic	Haldol Zyprexa Seroquel	haloperidol olanzapine quetiapine
Antidepressant	Elavil Tofranil Sinequon Paxil	amitriptyline imipramine doxepin paroxetine
Anti-seizure	Tegretol Trileptal	carbamazepine oxcarbazepine
Gastrointestinal	Lomotil Librax Bentyl Imodium Phenergan Zantac	diphenoxylate and atropine chlordiazepoxide dicyclomine loperamide promethazine ranitidine
Motion Sickness	Transderm-Scop	scopolamine

Category	Brand Name	Generic Name
Muscle relaxants	Transderm Flexeril Robaxin Norflex Zanaflex	scopolamine cyclobenzaprine methocarbamol orphenadrine tizanidine
Vertigo	Bonamine	meclizine

As with other dementogens, the cumulative effect sets the stage for Alzheimer's and dementia. Not only is it the negative cumulative effect of time but also from taking several anticholinergic medications at a time.[3]

The bottom line: if you are age sixty-five or older and taking anticholinergic medications, make sure you are off within three to six months at the maximum, or switch to one with low anticholinergic activity. There are better ways to treat these illnesses than medications that cause Alzheimer's and dementia.

CHAPTER 9

DEMENTOGEN 4: TOO MUCH COPPER

COPPER IS AN essential mineral, which is why I didn't include it with the other heavy metals in dementogen 1. It is generally not harmful like mercury, lead, arsenic, and cadmium unless you are consuming too much of it. Your body needs copper, but not too much.

Tap water often contains copper from pipes, and generally speaking, foods that contain copper include shellfish, seeds, nuts, organ meats, wheat-bran cereals, whole-grain products, and chocolate.[1]

IT'S A FACT

Zinc deficiency is very common in those age sixty-five and older. About 30 percent of the elderly are deficient in zinc.[2]

According to the US Department of Agriculture (USDA), here, in descending order from most copper to least, are common dietary sources of copper:

- apples
- asparagus
- avocado
- baking chocolate
- beef liver
- cashew nuts
- cereals (Cream of Wheat)
- chickpeas

- crab
- dark chocolate
- figs
- milk
- millet
- mushrooms
- oysters
- pasta (whole wheat)
- potatoes
- salmon
- sesame seeds
- spinach
- sunflower seeds
- tofu
- tomatoes
- turkey giblets
- yogurt[3]

With so many sources of copper, including vitamins and supplements, you might wonder how we could be low in copper, and it's true that people are seldomly deficient in copper.

We usually have more than enough copper in our bodies. So when is copper a dementogen? The answer may not be all that surprising: copper becomes a dementogen usually when you are older (over age sixty-five) and your body has insufficient zinc to maintain an approximate 1-to-1 copper-to-zinc ratio.

IT'S A FACT

Hot water causes more copper to be released from copper pipes than cold water. Let the water run for sixty seconds and drink cold water to minimize copper, or get a reverse osmosis water filter that removes about 98 percent of copper.

Too much copper is seldom a problem because our bodies balance the excess copper with zinc. We can ingest excessive copper from supplements containing copper, water contaminated with excessive copper, or fungicides containing copper sulfate. The RDA, or recommended daily allowance, for copper is 0.9 milligrams for adults. The normal range for copper in the blood is 85–180 mcg/dL. I recommend a range of 90–110.

But zinc intake usually decreases as we age, and our zinc levels drop. From no problem to a big problem, too much copper starts to cause damage (free radicals, inflammation, plaque buildup in the brain, cellular communication issues, and more) when you have too little zinc in your body.[4]

If you are wondering if you should increase your zinc levels, that is probably correct. As you age, your zinc levels usually drop.

IT'S A FACT

Wilson's disease is a rare genetic disorder that causes copper to accumulate in your liver, brain, and other organs.

A blood test will give you your zinc levels. I recommend serum zinc levels be 90–110 mcg/dL. A serum zinc level of 100 mcg/dL is a good goal, with a serum copper level of 100 mcg/dL, which creates a copper-to-zinc ratio of 1 to 1. That is then 90–110 mcg/dL for your copper and zinc amounts.

Zinc supplements are readily available. For most people, 11–30 milligrams of zinc will help balance out their copper. I wouldn't recommend taking more than 50 milligrams of zinc per day except for short periods during a cold or flu. The daily value for zinc is 11 milligrams a day for men and 8 milligrams for women. If you desire to supplement with zinc, I recommend just 15 milligrams a day of a zinc supplement.

The average intake of zinc from foods and supplements is about 13 milligrams per day for women and 16 milligrams per day for men in the United States.[5] Foods high in zinc include oysters (which contain more zinc per serving than any other food), red meat, poultry, beans, nuts, crab, shrimp, and whole grains.[6]

On a side note, if you take proton pump inhibitors to deal with acid reflux, you should take zinc supplements. Proton pump inhibitors are notorious for lowering zinc levels, among other not-so-healthy side effects.

If you are taking proton pump inhibitors, then you will need extra zinc to cover what the medication is lowering as well as what you'll need to balance your copper levels.

Zinc supplements significantly reduce the danger of copper becoming a dementogen. Without zinc, too much copper will help push people (especially those ages sixty-five and older) toward Alzheimer's and dementia.

Thankfully, zinc is a pretty easy and inexpensive fix for excessive copper, along with lowering your intake of high-copper foods, avoiding copper supplements, and not drinking tap water from copper pipes, especially hot water.

CHAPTER 10

DEMENTOGEN 5: SWEETENERS AND SUGARS

Of the many artificial sweeteners out there, such as aspartame, sucralose (Splenda), saccharin (Sugar Twin and Sweet'N Low), and neotame (NutraSweet), aspartame is one of the most common.

How common? Aspartame is an ingredient in more than six thousand different processed foods! You name it, and it probably has aspartame in it. From chewing gum to desserts, yogurts to vitamins, toothpaste to salad dressings, and medicines to diet drinks, aspartame is everywhere![1]

With artificial sweeteners, as with most dementogens, it is the cumulative effect and high amounts that cause dementia and Alzheimer's. This holds true for all artificial sweeteners.

Aspartame, in particular, has been found to cause

- anxiety,
- cognitive impairment,
- depression,
- headaches,
- irritable moods,
- learning impairment,
- memory issues,
- migraines, and
- sleep impairment.[2]

IT'S A FACT

Aspartame is two hundred times sweeter than sugar, and sucralose is six hundred times sweeter than sugar.[3] *Thus, only a little bit is needed, but every little bit adds up.*

Remember back in high school science class when it was time to dissect a frog? The liquid those frogs are preserved in is called formaldehyde. When aspartame is consumed, it breaks down into aspartic acid, phenylalanine, methanol, and formaldehyde in your body and brain.[4] About 10 percent of aspartame is broken down into methanol in the small intestine. Most of the methanol is absorbed and rapidly converted to formaldehyde.[5]

There is absolutely nothing good about formaldehyde being in your brain cells! Formaldehyde can kill cells in your tissues and your brain, converting to formic acid, which is highly toxic.

Cognitive symptoms you certainly don't want, such as "deficits in complex attention, inefficient information processing, reduced executive functioning, slower processing speed, and long-term memory loss," are all a result of consuming aspartame.[6] Aspartame is poisonous to the brain, but its negative impact is multiplied when consumed with carbohydrates.[7]

What's already bad becomes even worse when insulin levels spike—and they will spike when you eat high-sugar and high-carb foods, such as doughnuts, cereal, pancakes with syrup, bread, white rice, most desserts, pasta, and countless other foods!

Is Sugar a Dementogen?

You may be wondering if sugar itself is a dementogen. You could certainly say it is for all the damage that sugar does to the body. But according to one lengthy study with thousands of participants, neither Alzheimer's nor dementia (nor strokes) were associated with sugar-sweetened beverages. However, these were associated with artificially sweetened beverages.[8]

I do call sugar a dementogen. Some even call it a poison. Either way, the more you see sugar as not your friend, the better your health will be. But in comparing artificially sweetened beverages to sugar-sweetened ones, the artificial ones are far worse.

We have for years been sold the idea that "sugar-free" is a good thing.

When artificial sweeteners are used, rest assured that they more than eclipse any health benefits from the lack of sugar.

IT'S A FACT

"Do not be deceived, God is not mocked; for whatever a man sows, that he will also reap. For he who sows to his flesh will of the flesh reap corruption, but he who sows to the Spirit will of the Spirit reap everlasting life" (Gal. 6:7–8).

One of the challenges with the brain is relying on sugar (glucose) for energy, and unlike other cells in your body, your "brain cells cannot convert fats or proteins into glucose, so they depend on daily glucose for optimal functioning and survival."[9] Your brain needs energy, just not in the artificial form.

There is more than enough glucose in what you eat or drink daily for your brain to function. It's not like you need to start taking in sugar to feed the brain. There is plenty of glucose in carbohydrates and starches on hand to go around.

Here are a few healthier, natural sweeteners that do not trigger Alzheimer's or dementia:

- erythritol
- monk fruit
- stevia
- swerve
- xylitol
- yacon syrup

IT'S A FACT

Side effects of sucralose (Splenda) that can potentially lead to memory loss:

» *kills beneficial bacteria in the gut*

- » *damages the gut and causes leaky gut*
- » *produces toxic compounds when heated*
- » *may cause weight gain*
- » *is associated with a greater risk of insulin resistance and type 2 diabetes*
- » *spikes insulin levels*

For Your Ongoing Health

If you cannot avoid artificial sweeteners, be they aspartame, sucralose (Splenda), saccharin (Sugar Twin and Sweet'N Low), or neotame (NutraSweet), the next best thing is to reduce your intake. Yes, that will probably be the end of drinking virtually all sugar-free soft drinks and eating certain foods, but you no doubt knew they weren't healthy for you anyway.

Though artificial sweeteners are a dementogen, they are simply one of the many dementogens that accumulatively cause Alzheimer's and dementia. What is the best thing you can do to protect yourself from Alzheimer's and dementia regarding sugar and artificial sweeteners? There are two answers.

1. Avoid artificial sweeteners and reduce or avoid sugar.
2. Know how sugar harms the brain.

When you know how sugar harms your brain, you are far more likely to make healthier decisions. This knowledge will help you avoid Alzheimer's and dementia because this knowledge will usually stick with you for the rest of your life!

Sugar and your brain work like this:

1. Sugar (be it from a carbohydrate, fruit sugar, starch, or other) converts to glucose in your bloodstream.
2. Excessive glucose attaches to proteins, forming advanced glycation end products, obstructing their work and aging your brain and body.

3. Your body produces insulin to lower the glucose levels.

4. Your body produces insulin-degrading enzyme (IDE) to break down the insulin so it does not lower your sugar levels too low.

This happens all the time in real life, especially with afternoon snacks at a coffee shop, a meal at a fast-food restaurant, or dessert after a hearty dinner. Substantial insulin spikes are required to lower the sugars in most foods/drinks consumed in the standard American diet. People who consume meals, snacks, drinks, and late-night munchies may have five or six insulin spikes a day or more.

IT'S A FACT

Zevia is a soda sweetened with plant-derived stevia leaf extract and available in fifteen flavors. It contains zero sugar and zero calories and is a much healthier alternative to diet and regular sodas. I personally use soda water, such as Sanpellegrino, and add a squeeze of lime or lemon. You can also add stevia to it if desired.

Now, the body is a wonderful creation, and every time there is an insulin spike, the multitalented IDE (insulin-degrading enzyme) comes in and balances everything out. So you might be thinking, "What's the problem?"

It's this little-known fact: the IDE in your body must choose between (1) breaking down insulin in your blood, and (2) breaking down amyloid plaques in your brain.[10] Your amazing IDE cannot do both. It either breaks down the insulin your body created to handle what you ate/drank, or it breaks down the amyloid plaques that build up in your brain—the very plaques that are ever-present in the brains of people living with Alzheimer's.

Here is another important fact about IDE that you must know: it will always break down insulin first. Is it a good idea to keep your IDE busy lowering insulin levels with an artificially sweetened beverage? I don't think so. Drink a glass of water. Or green tea. Or coffee. Let your IDE stick to the most important things, such as breaking down those amyloid plaques!

IT'S A FACT

The brain binds up toxins in amyloid plaque to keep it from damaging the brain's neurons. But if you are not expelling plaque because your insulin-degrading enzyme (IDE) is busy, you are storing toxins in your brain.[11]

Another problem with insulin spikes is that high insulin triggers even more inflammation. Your body (and brain) need you to avoid insulin spikes. That's why lower-glycemic foods, fats, and fiber are so important and healthy. (We will discuss healthy food options later in this book.)

Now you know how sugar works with your brain. And you can never forget.

What's more, now you also know why the Alzheimer's and dementia epidemics are following right behind the diabetes epidemic, which is following the obesity epidemic. The excessive intake of sugars (in any form) ages and inflames our bodies and brains, and over time amyloid plaque in the brain cannot help but build up.

Avoid the dementogen of sweeteners, and lower your intake of sugary foods and beverages, and you will be well on your way to lowering your risk of Alzheimer's and dementia.

CHAPTER 11

DEMENTOGEN 6: ALCOHOL

THAT ALCOHOL CAN be bad for you is not a news flash for anyone, but that alcohol is also a dementogen may be.

Some argue that low to moderate alcohol consumption (two drinks a day for men and one drink a day for women), especially red wine and its high level of antioxidants, will lower your risk of cognitive decline.[1] But most research has found that alcohol increases your risk of cognitive decline.[2]

In my patients I've seen alcohol consumption lead directly to memory loss, brain atrophy, loss of sleep, and amyloid plaque buildup—not good at all, especially for those trying to reduce their risk of Alzheimer's and dementia.

In my opinion, it's best not to drink alcohol at all.

FIVE TIPS ON DRINKING

If you want to drink alcohol and simultaneously do all you can to minimize your risk of Alzheimer's and dementia, here are my suggestions:

1. Drink dry red wine. It's lower in sugar than other alcohols and higher in antioxidants.

2. Drink only small amounts, such as one 5-ounce glass.

3. Drink only a few times each week. Don't make it a daily habit.

4. Don't drink right before bed. It's bad for your metabolism, and it keeps you from going into a deep, restorative sleep.

5. If you have the ApoE4 gene (explained in chapter 5), it's best not to drink any alcohol at all.

You now know (from the previous chapter) how sugar boosts insulin levels, which then requires IDE (insulin-degrading enzyme) to balance out the insulin, and how the IDE has to focus on the insulin and ignore the rising amyloid plaque levels in your brain.

The dementogen of alcohol is just as dangerous, and then some. Mix it with the ApoE4 gene, and you are asking for trouble! For those with the ApoE4 gene, the negative effects of alcohol are multiplied.[3] What's more, the risk of getting Alzheimer's and dementia increases for ApoE4 carriers in proportion to the amount of alcohol they consume.[4]

IT'S A FACT

Many studies have found a connection between excessive alcohol intake and damage to the brain leading to dementia, deficits in learning, memory problems, mental disorders, and other forms of cognitive damage.[5]

Quite simply, alcohol is a dementogen, but for those with the ApoE4 gene, it's best to see alcohol as straight brain poison.

Getting tested for the ApoE4 gene is a good move, both for prevention and peace of mind, or you can use your parents' gene history (if you know it) to see if you carry the ApoE4 gene. Again, having the ApoE4 gene is no guarantee that you will get Alzheimer's or dementia, but drinking alcohol will only increase those odds.

If you choose to drink alcohol, please follow my five tips on drinking.

My ultimate recommendation is to avoid all alcohol consumption. Avoiding the dementogen of alcohol is easy, and not drinking alcohol will save you money and your brain. That's both cost-effective and good for your health!

CHAPTER 12

DEMENTOGEN 7: TRANS FATS

It's easy to hate bad fats. The problem with this dementogen is that trans fats are still in use even though they're so unhealthy that many countries have already banned their use (e.g., the United States banned artificial trans fats in 2015 with a deadline to eliminate them by 2018).

If you eat in a restaurant or shop at a grocery store, which we all do, then you have to be careful. Trans fats are hiding where you might not expect them, including in

- brownies,
- cakes,
- candies,
- canned frosting,
- caramels,
- chicken nuggets,
- chips,
- cookies,
- crackers,
- croissants,
- doughnuts,
- french fries,
- fried chicken,
- frozen pizza,
- ice cream,
- margarine,

- microwave popcorn,
- muffins,
- nondairy creamers,
- onion rings,
- pastries,
- peanut butter,
- pie crust,
- pies,
- refrigerated dough,
- salad dressings,
- shortening,
- Tater Tots, and
- vegetable oils.

If trans fats are listed in the ingredients, they're usually hiding behind words such as *hydrogenated fats* or *partially hydrogenated oil*. But here's the kicker: food manufacturers are not required to list trans fats on the label if they can keep the amount below 0.5 grams (500 milligrams) per serving. This means they can claim there are zero trans fats as long as it's below 0.5 grams per serving![1]

It's a complete lie, but unfortunately the "zeros" add up. You could be eating 500 milligrams here and 500 milligrams there while thinking you are avoiding trans fats entirely.

None of the foods listed previously are on any list of healthy things to eat, but still, the point is that trans fats are everywhere, and people are consuming trans fats without even knowing it. And that is bad news for their brains!

How Bad Are Trans Fats for Your Brain?

Online New Health Advisor has a quick take on trans fat that ought to be enough to scare almost anyone into avoiding it at all costs:

- Trans fat is the worst type of fat in food: it has no good properties, increases bad cholesterol, and lowers good cholesterol.
- This increases the risk of heart disease, stroke, high blood pressure, obesity, and more.
- Studies link trans fats to type 2 diabetes, liver problems, infertility, depression, Alzheimer's disease, breast cancer, and prostate cancer.

Regarding the brain, trans fats are linked to an increased risk of dementia. One study in Japan found those who consumed more trans fats had a significantly higher risk of getting Alzheimer's disease or dementia later in life. How much of an increased risk? A whopping 50–70 percent![2]

IT'S A FACT

Trans fats are found in many processed foods, especially in

- » *any processed food, fried or battered;*
- » *stick margarine and shortening; and*
- » *cakes, cake mixes, pies, pie crust, and doughnuts.*[3]

The brain, as you know, is about 60–70 percent fat. Trans fats have a nasty way of working into the brain cells and being incorporated within the cell membrane. As a result, the brain's cell membranes become stiff, distorted, and unable to pass nutrients back and forth effectively. Communication is disrupted, and your mental performance decreases—as you and your brain cells become partially hydrogenated! (The hydrogenation process allows oils to be hardened in stick form, such as stick margarine.)

Trans fats also increase inflammation in the brain. But that's not all. Not only does the damage from trans fats increase your risk of Alzheimer's and dementia, but that risk increases exponentially as you age.[4]

IT'S A FACT

If you have an ApoE4 gene, be extra careful, for the ApoE4 gene accelerates dietary fat absorption, increasing your cholesterol levels.[5]

Quite clearly, trans fats are bad for everyone, but like the other dementogens, the accumulative effect makes it much worse for the older population, especially those sixty and older.

The best recommended course of action is to avoid all foods that might potentially contain trans fats, whether they are listed on the label or not.

CHAPTER 13

DEMENTOGEN 8: GENERAL ANESTHESIA

When my mom fractured her hip several years ago, she already had mild dementia. They put her under general anesthesia for about two hours during the surgery, and her dementia had significantly worsened when she came out. It was as if years of memory loss had suddenly happened in those few short hours. She lost a lot of ground after her hip surgery. It was shocking to her and our family, but it is remarkably common.[1]

Looking back, I could have

- talked to her anesthesiologist to make sure her oxygen levels remained high and her blood pressure didn't go too low during surgery;
- put her on a choline supplement (cytidine choline or alpha-GPC choline supplements) after surgery to help with memory function and to increase acetylcholine in her brain, which supports memory;
- given her a glutathione supplement or a glutathione IV to help clear the anesthesia out of her body shortly after her surgery, when she was able to take supplements (see appendix F); and
- prescribed her a vasoactive intestinal peptide (VIP) nasal spray to help reduce inflammation in the brain.

I didn't know this at the time and couldn't do these quickly enough. But now that you know, you can. If you, your friends, or your family are over age sixty (especially over sixty-five) and need surgery requiring anesthesia, be aware, be careful, and be proactive.

IT'S A FACT

COVID-19 has been found to impair memory, cause stroke, and increase brain inflammation, which increases the risk of Alzheimer's and dementia.[2]

According to Dr. Dale Bredesen, multiple layers of danger are associated with surgeries requiring general anesthesia. You may not be able to avoid them completely, but you can minimize their impact as much as possible. Those dangers include

- anesthesia is usually toxic to the brain,
- anesthesia can cause hypoxia (poor oxygenation),
- anesthesia can cause hypotension (low blood pressure),
- surgery causes severe stress (cortisol levels rise),
- antibiotics given after surgery harm the gut, and
- inflammation from the surgery and the healing process is harmful to the body and the brain.[3]

These dangers have been found, as they did with my mom, to accelerate Alzheimer's and dementia symptoms. Even if you have no Alzheimer's or dementia to begin with, after a surgery that requires anesthesia, your risk of Alzheimer's and dementia just doubled if you are over fifty![4] As you would expect, the more times you go under general anesthesia and the longer you are under general anesthesia, the greater your risk of Alzheimer's and dementia.

If the surgery is optional, then I suggest that you opt out. But if it is needed, see if it can be done with local anesthesia. Spinal anesthesia is another option but is not much better than general anesthesia.[5]

If you can't opt out of the surgery and local anesthesia isn't an option (such as with most head, brain, chest, neck, or spinal surgeries), then apply as many of the following seven steps as you can.

1. Talk with the anesthesiologist beforehand to ensure high oxygen levels and normal blood pressure levels are maintained.

2. Look for ways to lower stress (cortisol levels) before and after surgery. See my *Stress Less* book for more information.

3. Don't take antibiotics any longer than necessary, and work to feed your gut healthy, probiotic foods or supplements afterward.

4. To reduce inflammation, eat anti-inflammatory foods and take anti-inflammatory supplements, such as curcumin (500 milligrams, one to two tabs twice daily) and omega-3 (1,000 milligrams twice daily). Some physicians have their patients wait one week before taking omega-3 supplements.

5. Take a glutathione supplement or IV to help clear the anesthesia out of your body. (See appendix F.)

6. Consider using a vasoactive intestinal peptide (VIP) nasal spray to help reduce brain inflammation.

7. Rest, sleep, and do light exercise after surgery when cleared by your doctor.

For younger people, general anesthesia is a lot less dangerous. It will usually have a minimal impact or no impact at all. But for older people, especially those sixty-five and older, general anesthesia should be avoided if possible.

Some people need multiple surgeries that require going under general anesthesia each time. Whatever their ages (and definitely if over age fifty), they should be following the previous seven steps, especially (1) watching their oxygen and blood pressure levels during surgery, and (5) clearing the anesthesia out of their bodies after surgery.

Strangely enough, the increased risk of Alzheimer's and dementia can continue for several years after general anesthesia. It's as if the anesthesia is still "in the system," even though it's not. Some bypass-surgery patients experienced a decline in their memory ability as much as five years after the surgery.[6]

Now, bypass surgeries are much more intense (stopping the heart, diverting blood to an artificial pump, and more) than many other surgeries that also require general anesthesia, but that makes prevention all the more important. I prefer that my cardiac patients have stents—which only use a sedative instead of general anesthesia—rather than bypass surgery, which always uses general anesthesia.

IT'S A FACT

Herbs that help lower cortisol levels include

» *ashwagandha,*

» *rhodiola,*

» *lemon balm, and*

» *chamomile.*[7]

When the brain has less oxygen than it should, brain cells die, which accelerates brain aging. That holds true for everyone, regardless of age.

Though general anesthesia is a dementogen, you will not often find yourself needing it. And that's a good thing! If you cannot avoid it, then be careful before and after. By doing so, you will significantly reduce the risk of anesthesia causing you any problems at all.

CHAPTER 14

DEMENTOGEN 9: MARIJUANA AND OTHER DRUGS

THAT MARIJUANA (CANNABIS) is a dementogen will surprise hardly anyone. We've known for decades that marijuana interferes with the brain.

Marijuana comes with a "bonus." According to the National Institutes of Health, frequent use of marijuana doubles your risk of developing schizophrenia in the future, and daily use increases the risk as much as five times.[1]

Randomly (though I'm sure it's genetic), it seems to flip a switch in some people's brains, making them schizophrenic for the rest of their lives. I can't tell you how many schizophrenic patients I've worked with over the years who used marijuana as a teen. They can now attribute their lifelong battle (almost always the case), ongoing medical expenses (always the case), and messed-up lives (almost always the case) to marijuana.

With marijuana there are a lot of questions, such as:

- Does the schizophrenic switch flip for everyone? No, it's random. But it's a risk that I would not recommend playing with. I know my many schizophrenic patients would agree.

- Is light use or heavy use of marijuana more dangerous? As with alcohol, heavy use is worse and more likely to cause brain damage. However, the switch to schizophrenia can be flipped by light or heavy use.

- What about using marijuana for medical needs? For treating chronic pain and intractable nausea, it has value. That's an OK use for marijuana—for the very small percentage of people who use it as such.

- Does marijuana really damage the brain? For most people who habitually use marijuana, it can cause brain damage.[2]
- What's wrong with the recreational use of marijuana? I can't answer the right/wrong question for people. All I can do is tell them the proven risks and results of using marijuana. They have the right and freedom to live the lives they want.

With all that said, if you want to strengthen your brain, avoid Alzheimer's and dementia, and live a long, healthy life, then marijuana is not your ticket. That applies to any drug, alcohol use, smoking, unhealthy eating, not exercising, and more.

With marijuana, there are a lot of choices to make, such as:

- Do you want to increase your risk of being schizophrenic? You don't know if you will be affected or not. The switch to schizophrenia is the luck of the draw.
- Do you want to increase your Alzheimer's and dementia risks substantially? Most Alzheimer's and dementia patients are ages sixty-five to eighty. I know teens think that they are invincible and nothing can hurt them, but they will someday be senior citizens. MRI scans of people (average age of sixty-seven) who used cannabis heavily when they were young (as teens and twentysomethings) showed they had smaller hippocampal memory centers than those who didn't use cannabis.[3] The brain always pays the price later.

IT'S A FACT

Anything you can do to strengthen the synapses in your brain will decrease your risk of Alzheimer's and dementia.[4]

- Do you have dreams and goals? Marijuana is the "lazy pill" or "slug drug." For most chronic users, it removes drive and ambition. As a result, chasing dreams, reaching your full potential, and career advancement are often never achieved.

- Do you want to be addicted? Marijuana is addictive. What's more, it's a known gateway drug that usually ushers in worse drugs.

- Do you want to make learning more difficult? Marijuana provides the brain with substantially less energy. Not only does this dull any desire to learn; it makes learning much more difficult. It has been found to have negative effects on the brain and educational outcomes, and these effects last longer than the temporary high.[5] My analogy is this: Walk in a straight line on a clear trail or through untamed underbrush full of vines, roots, rocks, and thorns, with the fastest one winning the prize. Which would you choose?

- Do you want a lower IQ? Those who use marijuana regularly have lower IQ scores than those who do not.[6] The rate of decline mirrors the amount of marijuana used. The more you use, usually the lower your IQ scores.

- Do you want to harm your brain? Chronic marijuana use has been found to impair memory, reduce the ability to process information, make recalling events more difficult, inhibit learning new info, decrease verbal and visual memory, and shorten attention.[7]

The dementogen of marijuana is easily avoidable, and doing so also saves you time, money, and a lot of wasted effort.

If you used marijuana when you were young, applying all the brain-friendly principles in this book will certainly help. Though brain cells that died from marijuana use are gone, the brain can mend itself in many ways.

THC Levels in Marijuana

Before the 1990s, the THC content of marijuana was less than 2 percent. Between 1995 and 2015, there was a 212 percent increase in the THC content in marijuana. In 2017 popular strains of marijuana contained a THC content of 17–28 percent in Colorado dispensaries. THC products are now concentrated, including THC oil dabs (concentrated forms of butane hash oil) and THC edibles, such as THC oil gummies. These products have THC concentrations as high as 95 percent.[8]

Human studies have shown that long-term use (greater than ten years) and heavy use (greater than five joints a day) of cannabis resulted in bilaterally reduced hippocampal volumes and significantly worse performance on verbal learning. Significant brain development occurs in adolescence, and long-term or heavy marijuana use can reduce the size of the hippocampus, which is critical for learning and memory.[9]

Other Drugs as Dementogens

Many drugs are associated with cognitive decline. Long-term cigarette smokers are at an increased risk of cognitive impairment and possibly dementia. Smoking also increases plasma homocysteine levels, and elevated homocysteine levels are associated with increased Alzheimer's and dementia.[10]

Middle-aged cocaine-dependent individuals have psychological and physiological changes associated with old age, including cognitive decline, brain atrophy, and immune deficiency.[11]

Amphetamines include crystal meth, methamphetamine, and MDMA (often called Ecstasy or Molly). There are also prescription amphetamines, including Adderall, Desoxyn, Dexedrine, Dynavel, Evekeo, ProCentra, and Vyvanse.

A recent study looked at patients with amphetamine-related disorders that included both amphetamine use disorder and amphetamine-induced psychotic disorder and found that these patients may have nearly five times the risk of developing Alzheimer's and other types of dementia.[12]

Not all drugs appear to be damaging to the brain, and two look promising to increase cognition. Research is now being conducted using psychedelic drugs: psilocybin and LSD in microdosing to treat Alzheimer's disease.

These psychedelic drugs "enhance functional neuronal connectivity, stimulate neurogenesis, restore brain plasticity, decrease inflammation, and enhance cognition." The ideal dose for cognitive enhancement and the dosing frequency cannot be determined until more research is done.[13]

When it comes down to it, avoiding the use of marijuana and other drugs is the best measure to decrease your risk of Alzheimer's and dementia.

CHAPTER 15

DEMENTOGEN 10: CHRONIC INFECTIONS

Chronic infections, which are long-lasting or recurrent, are a dementogen. Why? Because chronic infections are associated with chronic inflammation, which directly increases the risk of Alzheimer's and dementia, in addition to many other diseases.

IT'S A FACT

Floss your teeth. One of the best ways to fight periodontitis (gum disease) is the simple act of flossing your teeth once or twice daily.[1]

Typically, chronic infections can last for many years, all the while hiding from your immune system. The symptoms may have gone unnoticed or been no big deal to start with, but their persistence should be a warning, such as chronic

- abdominal bloating,
- cold symptoms,
- cough,
- diarrhea,
- earache,
- fatigue,
- fever blisters,
- hoarseness,
- joint pain,
- low-grade fever,

- muscle aches,
- sensitive tooth or teeth,
- shortness of breath,
- sinus congestion,
- sore or bleeding gums, or
- sore throat.

These are all simple signs that something might be wrong.

Chronic infections are often viral or bacterial. You somehow caught it, but your body didn't get rid of it fully. Believe it or not, every adult usually carries several chronic infections around with them! Some last for months, and some for years.

The worst thing is that we seldom stop long enough to do something about them. We say we can "put up with" the sniffles, cough, fatigue, or whatever the symptom might be, but it's not good for our health. Even worse is that as we age, these chronic infections may increase in severity and cause more damage. For those age sixty-five and older, it's the peak time.

I see it all the time with my patients.

But this is where things take a turn for the worse. As you know, the brain always pays for it later; that is exactly what happens! The increased inflammatory load of these chronic infections on an aging population is causing the amyloid plaque buildup that accompanies Alzheimer's and dementia.[2]

That chronic infections lead directly to plaque in the brain and increase the risk of Alzheimer's and dementia is a good enough reason to address that pesky cough or other "minor" ailments that never seem to go away.

Common Chronic Infections

Of the many chronic infections that come through my office doors, these are the most common:

- chronic bronchitis
- chronic ear infections
- chronic fatigue (often the West Nile virus or the Epstein-Barr virus, or EBV, which is part of the Herpes family of viruses)

- chronic sinus infections
- cold sores (herpes virus HSV-1)
- COVID-19 (the long-term type)
- gum inflammation (gingivitis)
- Lyme disease (a bacterial infection) and coinfections
- serious gum disease (periodontal disease)

There are many other infections, but these are the most common ones for my patients.

The constant inflammation from chronic infection causes damage to the body, creates plaque in the brain, and thereby increases the risk of Alzheimer's and dementia.

How do you know? Symptoms give it away usually, but also you can check your blood. Quite often, blood work will reveal infections that you didn't even know you had.

IT'S A FACT

Thymosin alpha 1 is a peptide that stimulates your T cells to find and eliminate viruses, and it helps your immune system become stronger and more resistant to viral infections. Thymosin alpha 1 is an injection usually given two times per week and is prescribed by a medical doctor. (This peptide is now difficult to obtain due to new government regulations.)

Treating Chronic Infections

Usually, once you know what you are fighting against (from your blood work), it's pretty easy to boost your immune system and kill chronic infections with

- immune-boosting supplements such as the amino acid lysine 1000 milligrams three times per day to treat cold sores and 1000 milligrams one time per day to prevent them;

- a healthy lifestyle;
- healthy habits (such as flossing and brushing your teeth two to three times a day);
- healthy eating habits (refer to my book *Beyond Keto*);
- antibiotics, herbs, antivirals, or nano-silver solutions (such as Silver Biotics, not colloidal silver)—Silver Biotics nasal spray for chronic sinus infections, Silver Biotics nebulizer treatments for chronic lung infections, and Silver Biotics solution for infected gums (you can also use other nano-silver solutions);
- probiotics and prebiotics to restore beneficial bacteria to your gut;
- thymosin alpha 1 (see "It's a Fact" sidebar in this chapter) for chronic viral infections, or an oral thymus peptide such as Vladonix; and
- glutathione-boosting supplements or IV. Glutathione has powerful antiviral properties. (See appendix F.)

This process can take from a few weeks to several months. And if you are working on more than one chronic infection, it may increase the overall length of time a little bit. I've seen patients with several chronic infections, such as Lyme disease or Lyme disease coinfections, take one to three years or longer to clear everything out of their systems.

IT'S A FACT

Herpes viruses, including herpes simplex virus type 1 and varicella zoster virus (which causes shingles), have been implicated in the development of Alzheimer's disease. Antiviral treatment has been suggested to protect against the development of dementia in individuals infected with herpes.[3]

Thankfully, your body is more than happy to get rid of the chronic infections, and you will usually experience only mild to minimal symptoms from the medication or treatment as long as you follow a low-sugar, low-carb, healthy keto or Mediterranean diet and take adequate probiotics and prebiotics.

IT'S A FACT

It is estimated that 10 percent of cancers arise from viral infections.[4]

IT'S A FACT

Nutrients with antiviral properties include

- » *zinc,*
- » *vitamin C,*
- » *quercetin,*
- » *N-acetylcysteine,*
- » *elderberry, and*
- » *vitamin A (retinol, not beta-carotene).*

Here's another reason to take chronic infections seriously and to deal with them right away: some chronic infections have a "sleeping time bomb" relationship with Alzheimer's and dementia. Years, even decades, can go by from the initial infection to when the brain damage occurs.[5] The simple answer is to treat chronic infections right away.

Now that you know the top ten dementogens that harm your brain, it's time to create your plan for defeating them. This will include removing their effects from your body and avoiding or minimizing your exposure to them in the future. The next section of this book outlines my recommended plan to get you into the Healthy Brain Zone now and keep you there for life!

PART III:
THE HEALTHY BRAIN ZONE PLAN

DESPITE THE MANY dementogens that swirl around us, there are more than enough ways to block and overcome them. The following ten steps are proven, effective, and perfectly suited to be part of your daily life. They are all doable and easy to begin right now. There are always other steps that you might learn and incorporate over time, but these are some of the most impactful and beneficial. When it comes to preventing, slowing, managing, stopping, or reversing Alzheimer's and dementia, every step in the right direction counts as success and real progress. You are on your way!

CHAPTER 16

FORM YOUR PLAN

Knowing what's going on is vital for your brain and overall health. And when you know the facts, then and only then can you take the necessary steps to achieve the health you want.

Taking action is the whole reason for knowing what's going on. Whether it's a national health trend, a symptom you've noticed in your body, or a detail that makes everything run smoother, it's all important. Please don't ignore it.

As you formulate your plan to improve your brain health, there are many details to consider. This chapter outlines a great starting point for anyone, regardless of age, who wants to decrease the risk of Alzheimer's and dementia to the point that it's no longer a concern.

IT'S A FACT

Research suggests that almost everyone with Alzheimer's has insulin resistance in the brain.[1]

Get Your Blood Work

You can't form an effective plan if you don't know where you're starting. To know where you're starting in the fight against Alzheimer's and dementia, you have to know your numbers. That's why I usually recommend patients begin with a full panel blood test to figure out where they are currently. Then when you get the results back, you will know more clearly which areas need to be worked on.

I've provided a complete list of tests and your target values for each test in appendix A of this book. Please photocopy this appendix to show the doctor who orders your blood work, and then use it to compare the target values with your blood work reports. If you have a positive ApoE4 gene test (the Alzheimer's gene), it will be especially important for you to achieve the target values for blood work and trophic factors from the list in appendix A.

Looking at the target values in appendix A right now without your blood work will be a little confusing, but trust me, it will make much more sense when you can compare your results with these numbers. Also, the first part of the book explains many pieces on this list to be tested, and when you finish the book, you will understand the rest. Knowledge is your power because the more you know, the better equipped you are to make the right health decisions for your current and long-term needs.

Get Other Testing

As I said, I believe everyone needs a full-panel blood test as a first step. That's because, regardless of our genetics, all of us need to monitor those numbers throughout our lives in order to prevent, fix, repair, or reverse the damage dementogens can cause. Beyond that, most should want to know their genetic risk level for developing Alzheimer's. If that's you, I strongly recommend the ApoE genetic (genotype) test I discussed in chapter 5 and following the dietary and lifestyle recommendations.

If you've noticed early signs of cognitive decline, please review chapter 3 to assess the level of progression for your symptoms. If you want more conclusive evidence of what you're dealing with, then consider getting one of the brain scans I discussed in that chapter.

In Alzheimer's cases, a positron emission tomography (PET) scan will show a consistent pattern of decreased glucose uptake,[2] especially in your hippocampus, which is located near your temples. The hippocampus is where information is stored temporarily before the brain processes it and moves it to your permanent memory.

Evaluate Your Test Results

The PET scan of the brain is optional, but not the blood work. Why? Because you can do everything you need to do to fight Alzheimer's and dementia with the blood tests I recommend in appendix A. Once you have your blood work results, you'll want to compare them to the target values I've listed in appendix A.

Your blood work results will determine your plan. Then you will know what steps from the following chapters are required to slow, manage, stop, or reverse memory loss and put you in the Healthy Brain Zone.

For the rest of this chapter, I'll highlight a few key blood test results to look for, and the rest of the chapters of this book will outline the twelve steps you need to follow in order to correct these numbers and put yourself on the path to the Healthy Brain Zone.

A1c and glucose levels

One of the most common dementogens is sweeteners and sugars (from sweets, carbs, and starches). Your hemoglobin A1c numbers will tell the story (an A1c number of 5.3 or lower is great, 5.7–6.4 is prediabetic, and 6.5 or higher is diabetic). About 40 percent of the adult US population is diabetic or prediabetic. People with type 2 diabetes may be two times more likely to develop Alzheimer's.[3] So if you have type 2 diabetes or are prediabetic, now is the time to take action.

Even if your A1c and glucose levels are normal, keep an eye on your waistline. Those with more belly fat have an almost three times greater risk of dementia than less-overweight people.[4] In light of this, losing weight is a great part of your action plan.

But don't lose too much! You need to maintain a minimum body mass index of 18.5 if you're a woman and 19.0 if you're a man if you are under age sixty-five, but higher if you are over sixty-five. Losing too much weight increases the risk of sarcopenia (loss of muscle) and osteopenia (loss of bone). People with these diseases have an increased risk of cognitive decline.[5]

A healthy keto diet will help. (You've probably heard of the ketogenic diet, or the keto diet for short: a low-carbohydrate, high-fat, and moderate-protein eating plan. However, there is a healthy keto diet and a very unhealthy one. Many people on the keto diet are following an unhealthy version of the diet. That's why throughout this book you'll notice I will specify eating a "healthy keto diet." A healthy keto diet includes a lot of healthy fats, and I explain more about this in chapter 25.)

IT'S A FACT

Your brain works hard! The 500 trillion synapses (neuron cell connections that communicate back and forth) in your brain are always busy. Your brain uses 20 percent of your body's total energy supply even though it's just 2 percent of your total body mass.

Cholesterol levels

Your blood work results will include your cholesterol numbers. Everyone is told to lower their cholesterol, but it is worth noting that if you push it below 150, you may be starving your brain and increasing your risk of brain atrophy.[6] A cholesterol level between 150 and 200 is best for your brain.

Chronic infections and inflammation

If your blood test shows that you have elevated hs-CRP that doesn't come down, this may be an indicator of chronic infections or Lyme disease. All chronic infections increase the risk of cognitive decline, whether you know you have them or not. Standard blood work will not usually confirm if you have chronic infections, which is why I recommend specific blood work for Lyme or Lyme coinfections, antibodies to herpes simplex virus 1, and more. Please compare your results with the target values in appendix A.

Inflammation also causes cognitive decline. Remember, type 1 Alzheimer's is usually associated with elevated inflammatory markers, including an elevated C-reactive protein, an increase in tumor necrosis factor, an increase in interleukin-6 (IL-6), or an increase in nuclear factor kappa B (NFKB). It is also associated with a decrease in the albumin-to-globulin ratio.

Don't Put It Off!

These key blood work results, along with indicators of suboptimal nutrient and hormone levels and toxins in the body, will paint the full picture of where you're starting. And the time to start is now! A list of the most important blood tests is in appendix A.

Please don't delay. The first phase of Alzheimer's and dementia is when communication between brain cells is jammed, connections are lost, and cells die. The best time to take action is now. Beware of anyone, especially a doctor, who tells you to wait, see how it is, and come back next year. When most people are diagnosed with Alzheimer's or dementia, it's already been affecting them for fifteen to twenty years![7] The earlier you take action, the better off you are.

Never forget that Alzheimer's and dementia are not hopeless or inevitable. The scary statistics, such as the rate of new Alzheimer's cases doubling every five years from age sixty-five to ninety,[8] are based on people who are doing nothing to prevent, slow, manage, stop, or reverse memory loss.

They are not taking action, but you are. Every step is a positive movement, moving toward a better and stronger brain. Every step, even if it feels small and insignificant, is a step in the right direction. You are taking action, so be encouraged. You are on the right road!

The remaining chapters in this book outline the twelve steps of the Healthy Brain Zone plan that will benefit everyone, whether they have no memory loss and are being entirely preventive or have early, late, or even severe memory loss.

For most people these twelve steps will be all they need to slow, manage, stop, or reverse memory loss. But if you need more, now that you know your brain and you know your numbers, you are armed with the exact details of where you are and where you want to go.

CHAPTER 17

STEP 1: BREAK INSULIN RESISTANCE

THE VAST MAJORITY of patients with Alzheimer's or dementia are insulin resistant. Clearly then, you must not let your brain or body become insulin resistant!

The opposite of insulin resistance is insulin sensitivity. That is the goal, but like a pendulum, it can only be achieved by swinging away from insulin resistance and toward insulin sensitivity.

IT'S A FACT

The ApoE4 gene interferes with your body's ability to use insulin properly. The result: your brain cells are starved for glucose.

This statement immediately makes my patients ask:

- What exactly is insulin resistance?
- Can I reverse it?
- Will my insulin sensitivity come back?
- How long will it take?

All are good questions. In the *Beyond Keto* and *Dr. Colbert's Hormone Health Zone* books, I go into greater detail about insulin resistance, but here is a synopsis, broken into several points.

INSULIN RESISTANCE: TYPE 3 DIABETES

Everyone has heard of type 1 and type 2 diabetes, but there is a less-known type 3 diabetes, which is diabetes of the brain. That is because this form of diabetes is associated with Alzheimer's disease. Type 3 diabetes is not an officially recognized health condition yet, but many have started referring to Alzheimer's with this moniker. When a brain is severely insulin resistant, that person has type 3 diabetes and their brain cells simply cannot take in sugar adequately.

Insulin Resistance: What Is It?

As you eat, your body produces insulin to manage and lower your sugar levels (from carbs, starches, and sugars in the food you eat) while simultaneously converting that sugar to energy that you burn or store (as fat). But over time, the repetitive pumping of excessive amounts of insulin (as a direct result of the typical high-carb, high-sugar diet) makes the cells resistant to insulin so that cells in your body and brain cannot take in sugar (glucose) easily from your blood. Eventually, the insulin resistance worsens, and the brain will be starving for fuel. The microscopic insulin receptors on the cell membrane of all cells (including brain cells) work less efficiently, so the body produces even more insulin to do its job, but with ever-decreasing effectiveness.[1] That is insulin resistance, and it typically gets worse with age.

The number of insulin receptors on a cell membrane varies from 40 on red blood cells to 200–300x10^3 for adipocytes (fat cells) and hepatocytes (liver cells).

Insulin Resistance: Signs and Symptoms

Here are some of the most common signs and symptoms of insulin resistance:

- A1c greater than 5.7
- belly fat—a waist measurement of 40 inches or more in men and 35 inches or more in women
- a body mass index greater than 25
- fasting glucose levels greater than 114
- fasting insulin levels greater than 5.5
- an inability to fast
- low-blood-sugar episodes[2]

IT'S A FACT

The leading causes of memory loss are insulin resistance, prediabetes, and type 2 diabetes, all of which are preventable and reversible.[3]

Insulin Resistance: Weight Gain

Insulin resistance will ruin your weight loss plans. Your body cannot adequately burn fat if you eat too many carbohydrates. That is because the high insulin levels, which are required to counterbalance the high-carb foods, stop your body's fat-burning mode and trigger fat storage mode instead. Belly fat is the typical result.

Insulin Resistance: Rising Sugar Levels

When insulin is no longer effective or efficient, blood sugar levels rise in the bloodstream. That is what a hemoglobin A1c level measures. Someone with an A1c of 5.7–6.4 is prediabetic and diabetic if 6.5 or higher. Your goal is to have your A1c even lower, preferably below 5.3.

IT'S A FACT

Insulin Resistance and the ApoE4 Gene: For those with the ApoE4 gene, insulin resistance happens more quickly, starting as early as their teens. They cannot take sugar (glucose) into the brain cells as well, and if they eat the normal high-carb diet, the insulin resistance is exponential.

Insulin Resistance: The Worst Foods

You can protect your brain by avoiding foods that spike blood sugar levels, as those foods also spike your insulin levels, and insulin spikes are bad for the brain. The worst are foods such as bread, potatoes, and white rice, as they are absorbed more quickly. The next worst are foods with lots of sugar, such as candy, ice cream, and cakes.[4] The answer is to eat foods that don't spike your insulin levels.

Insulin Resistance: Where It Leads

Insulin resistance is the root cause of virtually every chronic disease, including obesity, prediabetes, type 2 diabetes, heart disease, many cancers, Alzheimer's, and dementia. Sadly, insulin resistance affects 88 percent of the US population, and nine out of ten people are unaware.[5] Insulin resistance also causes inflammation, which is destructive to the brain and body and is associated with autoimmune diseases.

Insulin Resistance: Exercise Helps

Increasing the size of your muscles will help reverse insulin resistance and improve insulin sensitivity. I have even seen muscle-building stop and even reverse type 2 diabetes, especially when combined with a healthy keto diet. That is because muscles burn sugar, thereby decreasing the amount of insulin required to manage the food you've eaten.

Insulin Resistance: Balanced Hormone Levels Help

Optimizing hormone levels can also play a big part in improving insulin sensitivity. I have helped many patients balance their hormone levels, which in turn helps reverse osteoporosis, prevents and reverses sarcopenia, and helps increase even more muscle mass, which all compound to help further improve insulin sensitivity.

Insulin Resistance: How to Reverse It

The most effective and only long-term way to reverse insulin resistance and regain insulin sensitivity is to stop or dramatically decrease the consumption of high-sugar foods (carbs, starches, and sugars). This decreases your body's need to produce insulin, automatically lowering your blood sugar levels. And that, by the way, is also the best way to prevent and treat type 2 diabetes and prediabetes!

Insulin Resistance: The Right Diet Will Help

The best diets to reverse insulin resistance are a healthy keto diet or a healthy Mediterranean-style diet (as outlined in my *Beyond Keto* book). These diets are low-carbohydrate, low-sugar, and high in healthy fat, which is necessary to restore insulin sensitivity.

Insulin Resistance: How Long Will It Take?

Reversing insulin resistance is not instant. Some medications do help with insulin resistance somewhat, but it usually requires you to take the necessary action steps (changing diet, exercising, balancing hormones, and more). It will have an immediate and positive impact that you will probably notice and feel, but it will take a little time to improve your insulin sensitivity. The weight loss, muscle toning, clearing of symptoms, and improved mental focus along the way will no doubt be enjoyed! For most people, I tell them to expect noticeable insulin sensitivity improvement in one to two months, but it may take three to six months. Many patients see a complete reversal within six to twelve months from insulin resistance to insulin sensitivity.

This progressive slide toward insulin resistance is happening on a global scale. And as you can very well understand, it is part of the same obesity and type 2 diabetes wave that is affecting millions upon millions of people every day.

But there is an additional sense of urgency in all this. You see, the more insulin in your body and brain, the greater your risk of Alzheimer's and dementia.

IT'S A FACT

You are probably insulin resistant if you are

- *a male with a 40-inch or greater waist, or*
- *a female with a 35-inch or greater waist.*

We discussed this previously, but it all comes into play at this precise moment. As your body produces insulin to counterbalance the glucose (carbs, starches, and sugars) from foods you eat, your body also produces an insulin-degrading enzyme (IDE) to remove the insulin from your body so that it doesn't lower your blood sugar levels too low. If your blood sugar goes too low, you may experience blacking out, fainting, seizures, confusion, weakness, shaking, sweating, dizziness, fast heartbeat, and more, which are symptoms of hypoglycemia or low blood sugar.

IDE also has another major function. It breaks down the amyloid plaque associated with Alzheimer's and dementia.

Because the IDE must choose between breaking down the excessive insulin in your blood or breaking down the damaging amyloid plaque in your brain, you are fueling Alzheimer's and dementia by being insulin resistant.

Why? Because this enzyme is programmed to break down insulin first. And that means you are running out of time.

That is the sense of urgency!

Quite simply, every day, week, month, or year that you are insulin resistant is that much time you are forcing your IDE to choose between harming your body or harming your brain, and you know what the choice will always be: both will suffer.

And if that is not enough, your brain is more sensitive to or affected by insulin resistance than your body. What does that mean? If your body has a *little* insulin resistance, your brain usually has a *lot* of insulin resistance.

That translates into a hurting, sluggish, and starving brain, especially for those with the ApoE4 gene, leading to the formation of much-dreaded plaques and tangles that accompany Alzheimer's and dementia.

Look around. Everyone with belly fat, obesity, prediabetes, or type 2 diabetes is usually also insulin resistant! And insulin resistance increases with age, which harms the brain all the more.

The only way to prevent or break the cycle and rescue your brain from this downward spiral is to become insulin sensitive again. The only way to do that is by eating foods that do not cause insulin spikes. Yes, that will mean you will need to eat differently than those on the typical high-carb diet, but you certainly don't want to be part of the national health trends anyway.

DR. COLBERT'S HEALTHY BRAIN ZONE

The vast majority of patients with Alzheimer's and dementia are insulin resistant. But you have an advantage! This book is your recipe for Alzheimer's-free and dementia-free living! My book *Beyond Keto* goes into even more detail to help you break free of insulin resistance.

The way I see it, keeping the brain sensitive to insulin is one of the best insurance policies in the world.

CHAPTER 18

STEP 2: REMOVE TOXINS

TOXINS COME IN many different shapes and sizes. In fact, all of the dementogens discussed in part 2 of this book are toxic. But even though they are many, there are just as many things you can do to eliminate the toxic toll in your body and brain. Here are a few ideas:

Switch to natural cleaning products.

You don't have to purchase products full of chemicals to clean your home. Lemon juice is a great deodorizer, glass cleaner, and stain remover from aluminum, clothes, and porcelain. It can also bleach fabric if used with sunlight.

Vinegar can dissolve mineral deposits and grease, remove soap scum, mildew, and wax buildup, polish some metals, and deodorize. It can also clean brick and stone and some carpets. Use it to clean your coffee maker, shine windows, and deodorize your washing machine. A simple all-purpose cleaner can be made from four tablespoons of baking soda dissolved in one quart of warm water.

If you do use chemically-based cleaners, be sure to wear rubber gloves to keep the chemicals away from your skin so they are not absorbed into your body. Also be sure the room is well-ventilated so the fumes to do affect your lungs.

Use clean beauty and personal care products.

Many companies today are committed to offering chemical-free beauty products for your hair, skin, body, and more. You no longer need to apply personal products to your hair, face, and body that contain chemicals such as ammonia, formaldehyde, triclosan, parabens, phthalates, and aluminum chlorohydrate.

IT'S A FACT

Consuming artificial sweeteners results in insulin release from the pancreas, eventually leading to insulin resistance.[1]

Eat more fiber.

The colon is the body's most important toxin disposal system. It was designed to take out the trash on a daily basis, not once a week. But when it's constipated, like a backed up septic tank, the waste sitting in your colon and rectum can seep into your body and theoretically cause autointoxication, which is defined as a state of being poisoned by toxic substances produced in the digestive tract and especially in the colon. Proteins putrefy, carbohydrates ferment, and fats rancidify. In other words, the body becomes toxic from its own waste.[2]

You need twenty-five to thirty-five grams of fiber a day to keep the colon moving those toxins along. And remember, fiber and water work together to stimulate the colon. When you eat more fiber, make sure you drink more water. Your goal should be to have one or more bowel movements a day.

Eat clean, alkaline-forming foods.

Organic is always best. And even if you buy organic, make sure you wash your produce thoroughly. And try to have a diet that consists of at least 50 percent alkaline-forming foods, which include most fruits, green vegetables, lentils, spices, herbs and seasonings, and seeds and nuts. Limit your intake of meat and dairy, and always choose the leanest cuts of meat as possible.

IT'S A FACT

Fiber helps remove toxins from your body.[3]

Go ahead and sweat it!

Sweating and taking care of your skin can help your body get rid of toxins. Arsenic, cadmium, lead, and mercury can be released through your sweat in rates that match or even exceed urinary excretion in a twenty-four-hour period.[4] If you don't sweat, you're not fully healthy. So don't be afraid to perspire when you exercise or do yardwork. Aerobic exercise will increase lymphatic flow threefold, which means your body will release three times the amount of toxins.

Hop in the sauna.

If you don't work outdoors or for some reason you cannot exercise, talk to your doctor about sauna therapy. Infrared saunas use an infrared radiant heat that causes your body to eliminate up to three times more toxins than conventional saunas. Infrared sauna therapy enables one to release the toxic metals mercury, arsenic, lead, and cadmium in their perspiration.

Brush your skin.

If the pores in your skin become clogged with dead skin cells, the toxins may remain locked inside your body, putting more stress on your liver and kidneys. Dry-skin brushing for five minutes prior to taking a shower is an excellent way to keep your pores open and clear so that your skin is able to breathe and excrete toxins. A loofah sponge or natural soft-bristle brush is all you need. Start with the soles of your feet and work your way up to your neck, avoiding your face. Use firm, hard strokes to increase blood flow.

Clean the air.

Your lungs are exposed to many different environmental toxins. You have no choice but to breathe, and sometimes you can't avoid secondhand smoke, smog, car exhaust, dust, and other airborne trash. Here are a few ideas to get you started on the road to cleaner air in your home.

- Open a door or window and turn on a fan, provided you don't live next to a busy highway or street. On days with high pollen counts, keep windows closed and use the air conditioner.

- Replace your air conditioner's filter every two months, and clean your heating and air conditioning ducts at least every five years.

- If you have pets, keep them out of your bedroom when you sleep. It's best to keep all pets outdoors if at all possible.
- Avoid air fresheners that contain pesticides or are petroleum based. Stick with fragrance jars and dried botanicals. Or try essential oils such as lemon or lavender.
- Buy an air purifier for your bedroom. Hepa filters remove air particles with almost 100 percent efficiency. Ionizing air purifiers are also good at this.

Guard against common allergens and molds.

Consider buying encasements for your pillows, mattresses, and box springs to prevent dust mites, the most common cause of allergies. If dust allergies persist, consider replacing your carpets with hardwood floors or tile; take down drapes and buy non-fabric furniture. If your environment is humid, buy a dehumidifier. Guard against mold by watching for leaks in plumbing and the roof. Keep outdoor vegetation from touching your home. Ivy-covered walls may look beautiful, but those homes are much more susceptible to mold problems. Trim all bushes and trees to a foot away from your walls, and patch that roof before the next rainy season. If you have water stains on your ceiling or walls, you have mold and need to have it removed by professionals. Also, if you have a mildew odor in your home, you have mold and need to find the source and remediate it.

IT'S A FACT

People over sixty-five who have been taking anticholinergic medications for three or more years have a 54 percent higher risk of dementia.[5]

Removing Toxins From Your Body and Brain

Every known dementogen needs to be minimized, avoided, and removed from your body and brain. If you know it's bad for you, out it goes! This is vital in your effort to prevent, slow, manage, stop, or reverse Alzheimer's and dementia. When you remove toxins from your body and brain, you are closing the door on Alzheimer's and dementia, which is a very good thing!

Whether you are young or old, removing toxins is one of the best forms of prevention. If you are battling Alzheimer's or dementia already, whether mild, moderate, or severe, removing toxins may prove to be a beneficial boost.

The very nature of a dementogen is that it causes Alzheimer's and dementia. It slowly and surely chips away at your defenses. But you can stop these dementogens in their tracks and regain your health.

Removing these toxins means getting rid of them and staying rid of them.

All this helps to repair your gut and detox the liver and kidneys, which are an integral part of your own body's detoxification process. The combined effect of toxic overload can prevent your body from detoxifying itself.[6]

Detox With the Master Cleanse

You may want to use a master cleanse periodically to help your body detoxify. There are many kinds available at health food stores. Here's a simple recipe to create one yourself: mix 2 tablespoons of freshly squeezed lemon juice, 1/10 teaspoon cayenne pepper (or less), and stevia (to taste) in 8 ounces of spring water. Drink eight to twelve of these 8-ounce glasses a day while abstaining from any other foods and beverages except water, laxative herb tea, peppermint tea, or chamomile tea.

Thankfully, when the toxins are reduced enough, your body will be able to continue with its own detoxification. The sooner you can make that happen, the better, for toxins left alone have a nasty habit of spreading to other parts of your body, which naturally undermines your overall health.[7]

Usually, the more toxins you have in your body, the worse it is on your cholesterol levels. Good HDL cholesterol levels usually go down. What's worse is these toxins may then cause your gut to convert one beneficial nutrient (choline) into a toxic version (trimethylamine), which quickly oxides and causes plaque buildup in your arteries![8]

Toxins cause harm at every turn. The best health move you can make is to get them out of your system and then avoid them entirely.

Without the oppressive weight of toxins, your body and brain can go back to doing what they do best, decreasing your risk of Alzheimer's and dementia all the more!

CHAPTER 19

STEP 3: QUENCH YOUR INFLAMMATION

INFLAMMATION IS YOUR body's immune response to harmful stimuli, such as pathogens (viruses, bacteria), toxic compounds, and more. It has long been known to be the root cause of many chronic diseases that come through a doctor's office door, including arthritis, heart disease, most cancers, almost all autoimmune diseases, Parkinson's disease, and especially Alzheimer's and dementia.

Why is inflammation so powerful? I believe inflammation is able to cause damage in so many people's lives for two simple reasons:

1. Inflammatory symptoms usually get a bandage, not a fix.
2. Inflammation is persistently damaging.

Neither reason is scary at first glance, but think of it this way: Suppose you have a water leak behind your upstairs shower. On the floor below, a watermark appears on one wall, and you paint over it. Problem solved. It's nothing that another coat of paint every few months can't cure!

But behind the drywall, the water damage spreads. Over time, you may have wood rot, ruined walls, and mold. And if the mold affects the health of those in your family, you could be looking at costly medical bills, remediation of the home, and maybe even needing to sell your home. Clearly, it would have been better to fix the problem.

In the very same way, inflammation goes on below the surface. It slowly but surely causes more and more damage. The symptoms appear small and may even be in one specific area at first. We may try to treat them, but if the treatment is not a true fix, then it's just a patch.

Inflammation leads to disease *eventually*, not *immediately*. If all you do is put a bandage on it, you could be in serious trouble. That is especially true (and incredibly sad) when it comes to the brain. The amyloid plaque buildup in the brain that pinpoints Alzheimer's and dementia is the result of inflammation! Those plaques are an inflammatory response, and continued inflammation in the body will keep on causing more amyloid plaque to accumulate in the brain.

As I mentioned earlier, most people diagnosed with Alzheimer's and dementia have had it for fifteen to twenty years beforehand. To be diagnosed with Alzheimer's or dementia, patients are almost always in the moderate-to-severe range. They could have done much more to fix, repair, or reverse it had they started working on it earlier.

Inflammation needs to be quenched. Whatever the inflammation, wherever it is, it needs to be stopped! So, whether inflammation causes plaque in the arteries, pain in the joints, rashes on the skin, buildup of amyloid plaque in the brain, or other damage to the body and brain, you can no longer accept bandages as treatment. You must get to the source of your inflammation.

IT'S A FACT

The number-one source of inflammation in our bodies is usually leaky gut. Unfortunately a leaky gut leads to a leaky brain, which is the pathway to Alzheimer's and dementia.

Let me share a little personal example. (It wasn't "little" at the time, but in comparison to the brain, you could call it little.) Many years ago, I had terrible psoriasis all over my body. I tried every lotion, potion, treatment, cream, and pill under the sun.

Nothing changed until I figured out, by food allergy tests and the process of elimination, that I was very sensitive to gluten, peppers, and tomatoes. These three, which I ate almost daily and actually craved, were causing incredible inflammation in my gut. For me, that translated into psoriasis on my skin.

It took me about five years to finally figure it all out, including repairing leaky gut and restoring beneficial bacteria in the gut, but I did! When the symptoms finally cleared up, it was an incredible relief! I've had no symptoms for many years, but I still make it a practice to avoid or very infrequently eat gluten, peppers, and tomatoes.

In the same way, when you fix whatever has been causing your inflammation, the symptoms will usually eventually clear up. They have to because you removed the point of inflammation. You went to the source and fixed the problem. You remove the thorn, and you will eventually heal.

For the sake of your brain, quenching any inflammation is always the best plan of attack. Elevated blood sugar and insulin resistance are also associated with inflammation.

The Source of Most Inflammation

Most people with inflammation already know it. They have tell-tale symptoms in various parts of their body. If you are unsure if you have inflammation in your body, look at your blood work. Your high sensitivity C-reactive protein (hs-CRP) is a good sign. It is on your blood work list in appendix A.

If your hs-CRP number is greater than 0.9 mg/dL, you have inflammation somewhere in your body. Usually, however, people can tell they have inflammation from their ongoing symptoms.

I also check homocysteine levels. If your homocysteine level is greater than 7 µmol/L, inflammation in the brain is also present. This is also on your blood work list in appendix A. Elevated homocysteine is associated with an increased risk of Alzheimer's and atrophy of the brain. If my patients are age fifty or older, I recommend they check both their hs-CRP and homocysteine levels.

IT'S A FACT

About 10 percent of the US population over sixty-five develop Alzheimer's, and about two-thirds of them are women.[1]

Many of the dementogens, such as exposure to toxins, excess alcohol, a lack of exercise, smoking, and chronic stress, can contribute to inflammation in your body.[2] The most common cause of chronic inflammation is leaky gut, which is caused by whole or partially digested food molecules, bacteria, and fragments of bacteria and other molecules that leak through the intestinal lining and enter the bloodstream and cause an inflammatory response.[3]

You can easily imagine a small molecule slipping into the bloodstream through microscopic holes in your intestine. That's exactly what was happening when I had psoriasis. The gluten, peppers, and tomatoes I ate were damaging my gut and creating more microscopic holes, and the subsequent inflammation was the direct result.

Now imagine the same thing happening in your brain! Molecules can, as a direct result of chronic inflammation in other parts of your body, drift through the blood-brain barrier. The blood-brain barrier prevents harmful substances from reaching the brain, but chronic systemic inflammation can cause changes in the blood-brain barrier. Toxins are then able to enter your brain! That is precisely why Alzheimer's patients have triple the number of these toxins in their blood than healthy people.[4]

Because the gut and brain are directly connected, any effort to help heal a leaky gut will also usually help the brain by reducing the buildup of amyloid plaque, which directly reduces the risk of Alzheimer's and dementia. This also plays a key role in the slowing, managing, stopping, or reversing of Alzheimer's and dementia!

A big part of the inflammation in the gut and brain is from bad bacteria that have grown out of control. We all have a certain amount of bad bacteria in our guts, along with good bacteria, but if the balance shifts (for various reasons, usually from antibiotics) and the bad bacteria gain the upper hand, it's bad news for your body and brain. If the bad bacteria are left in charge, they digest the food, resulting in toxins being released into your body and brain.[5]

Unfortunately the bad bacteria in the gut increase the leakiness in the brain![6] Simply put, you don't want bad bacteria in control in your gut.

Steps to Restoring Your Gut

Restoring your gut so you can protect your brain from Alzheimer's and dementia requires three things.

1. Kill the bad bacteria in the gut with safe, natural supplements, not antibiotics. (See *Dr. Colbert's Healthy Gut Zone*.)
2. Restore a leaky gut immediately.
3. Restock your good gut bacteria immediately.

Doing so will usually have an immediate effect on the brain. And when you do this while also reversing your insulin resistance (chapter 17), you effectively stop damage to your brain on many levels!

I often tell my patients that having a healthy gut is one of their best defenses against Alzheimer's, dementia, and Parkinson's. Even if it may seem hard to believe, the gut and the brain are so closely impacted by each other, it's true.

The great naturopath Joseph Pizzorno has an excellent three-pronged protocol. These aren't steps you do one at a time; all three are to be done simultaneously to restore and repair a leaky gut.

1. Kill the bad bacteria—with oil of oregano or goldenseal root powder for at least one to two weeks and sometimes longer (four to six weeks). I prefer ADP tablets (oil of oregano) from Biotics Research for my patients, and I usually prescribe two before each meal for four to six weeks.

2. Restore the good bacteria—with multifactorial probiotics that include lactobacillus, Bifidobacterium, and multiple probiotic strains taken three times per day initially for one to two weeks, then one time per day thereafter, L glutamine (500 milligrams 1 capsule three times per day), quercetin (250 milligrams two times per day), and DGL (250–500 milligrams three times per day), fiber, prebiotics if needed, and other supplements if needed. I recommend continuing the probiotics and fiber after one month as well as the other supplements if needed. I also may add bone broth soup daily and other powerful probiotics and collagen if needed.

3. Stop damage going forward—don't repeat what caused the damage in the first place.[7]

The best long-term strategy for addressing a leaky gut and for keeping your gut healthy and whole (thereby directly benefitting your brain) is a diet that promotes and maintains a healthy gut. That's why I highly recommend a healthy keto diet. (I provide a deeper understanding of this type of eating in chapter 25 and in my books *Dr. Colbert's Healthy Gut Zone* and *Beyond Keto*.)

A healthy keto diet not only slows or stops inflammation, it also helps heal your gut, feeds your good bacteria, and protects your brain from plaque buildup. Basically, a healthy keto diet does it all!

IT'S A FACT

Cognitive decline is mostly the result of inflammation; a shortage of brain-boosting nutrients, hormones, other molecules; and toxic exposure.[8]

On a side note, one very common sign of inflammation is the presence of belly fat. Usually, the more belly fat someone has, the higher their inflammatory markers and the smaller their hippocampus (the brain's memory center). A shrinking hippocampus is not a good thing!

Also, belly fat itself is highly inflammatory. Inflammation may be caused by diet (as was my psoriasis), infections, toxins, a leaky gut, medications, or something else. Sugar and trans fats are inflammatory to everyone, and gluten and dairy are inflammatory to many.

But there is good news: when belly fat decreases, so does inflammation, which has exponentially good effects on your body and brain.

Everyone agrees that inflammation must be stopped because it leads directly to disease and often to Alzheimer's and dementia, but will they do anything about it? Sadly, not many will.

Most causes of inflammation are self-induced, and changing a habit, especially if it is a food and lifestyle habit, is not the easiest thing to do. But when it comes to the brain and the very real risk of Alzheimer's and dementia, making new habits is easy!

For every cause of inflammation, there are options and answers. If you have inflammation, don't ignore it, don't see how it is next year, and don't give it the bandage treatment. Find its root cause and fix it now. You will be very glad you did.

CHAPTER 20

STEP 4: PRACTICE INTERMITTENT FASTING

THE WORD *FASTING* does not get people very excited, but perhaps it should. You see, fasting is incredibly beneficial for your brain, not to mention benefitting your body in many other areas.

For most of my patients, adding intermittent fasting to their routine helped them get the health benefits they wanted and needed. I even had one patient with mild dementia get his job back as a result of intermittent fasting. His brain fog cleared up, and he regained his sharp mental focus after just three months of intermittent fasting.

That was a huge benefit for him! And yet practicing intermittent fasting cost him nothing. It's free.

Patients often ask me, "What exactly is intermittent fasting?" and "How will it help me?" Good questions. If you are wondering the same, I think you will like the answers.

Intermittent fasting is going without food between meals, such as twelve, fourteen, sixteen, or even twenty hours. The benefits of intermittent fasting are improvements in brain function, insulin sensitivity, energy levels, and weight loss.

This is where another question comes in: "How does intermittent fasting work?" This is the big one! Knowing the answer to this question has helped many patients "get it" and stay motivated to add intermittent fasting to their daily or weekly routine.

Here's how intermittent fasting works: The body breaks down the carbs and starches you eat into glucose and stores enough as glycogen to always have about twelve hours' worth on hand. It is *after* those twelve hours and *before* you eat again that intermittent fasting does its work. That is when the amazing happens!

After dinner, supposing you finish at 6 p.m., if you don't eat anything until breakfast the next morning at 8 a.m., those fourteen hours between meals count as intermittent fasting. But beware! Most people have snacks after dinner, and maybe even a late dessert or an early-morning glass of juice, which cancels intermittent fasting and its benefits.

When You Are Intermittent Fasting

When your body's store of glucose is used up (at around twelve hours since your last meal), it begins to do what you want and need it to do. Sometimes it's hard to believe how it works, but the body knows best. We just need to give it room to work its magic.

Here's what happens when you fast intermittently:

- Your metabolism usually shifts at around twelve hours, and you go from burning stored glucose to burning stored fat. Yes, the longer your intermittent fast, such as fourteen or sixteen hours, the more stored fat is burned off each time.
- Your risk of cardiovascular disease decreases due to the triglyceride fats being burned off.[1]
- Your insulin resistance goes down, and your insulin sensitivity goes up.[2]
- Your risk of type 2 diabetes decreases.[3]
- Your inflammation decreases everywhere.[4]
- Your blood pressure usually goes lower.[5]
- Your body produces the good protein brain-derived neurotrophic factor (BDNF) that strengthens the connections in your brain, principally those involved in memory and learning.[6]
- Your risk of Alzheimer's and Parkinson's decreases.[7]
- Your brain grows new nerve cells.[8]

- Your brain is protected from neurodegenerative disorders, Alzheimer's disease, and seizures.[9]
- Your brain is protected from amyloid plaque buildup.[10]

That is an incredible list! And to think that your body can do all this for you is equally amazing.

The fact that intermittent fasting helps to address many of the very issues involved in Alzheimer's and dementia, such as inflammation, insulin resistance, BDNF, nerve cell growth, plaque buildup, and more, is more than enough reason to practice intermittent fasting.

There is one more very important benefit of intermittent fasting that needs further explanation because of its specific value for those who are preventing or slowing, managing, stopping, or reversing Alzheimer's and dementia.

- Your body and brain "clean house" at the cellular level during intermittent fasting.

More specifically, intermittent fasting causes your body and brain to sweep out much of the cellular debris. This "trash" includes old cells, dead cells, denatured or damaged proteins and mitochondria, toxins, and the much-dreaded amyloid plaque and tangles. Worn-out cellular components, including mitochondria and proteins, are stripped of their building blocks to make new components for the cell.

You read that right: intermittent fasting also helps clear amyloid plaque out of your brain! Removing cellular debris helps restore the mitochondria (which are in every single cell in your body and brain). Interestingly, the mitochondria are tasked with producing adenosine triphosphate (ATP), and ATP is what your body uses for energy.

IT'S A FACT

Common sources of damage to your mitochondria: toxins, elevated blood sugar levels, inflammation, disease, some medications, and age.

In short:

- intermittent fasting removes cellular trash and recycles cellular components to make restored proteins and mitochondria
- removing cellular trash helps restore the mitochondria,
- restored mitochondria produce more ATP, and
- ATP gives you more brain energy, which usually translates to an improved memory.

I can't tell you how many patients (especially those in their sixties, seventies, and eighties) I've had over the years who come into my office with the same complaint: "I have no energy."

It's true. They have absolutely no energy. It's sad. And though energy production typically decreases as we age, having no energy is certainly not an option.

This whole process of cellular cleaning and increased energy is called autophagy, and it works amazingly well! I've had patients with no energy begin to practice intermittent fasting, and within a few short months, their energy levels rebound to the point that some don't know what to do with all their energy. Several had to start new hobbies, increase their exercise programs, or start a part-time job.

Your brain has a lot of mitochondria, so the refreshing and restoring of the mitochondria through autophagy will usually have a significant positive effect on your brain!

You can always use more energy and brain energy, can't you?

Your Intermittent Fasting Plan

The schedule you choose for your intermittent fasting is up to you. Maybe you will

- do the 14/10 plan: fasting for fourteen hours between dinner and breakfast; eating meals in a ten-hour window;

- do the 16/8 plan: fasting for sixteen hours between dinner and late breakfast/lunch; eating meals in an eight-hour window, which is one of the most popular plans and best for those with the ApoE4 gene;

- do weekdays: intermittent fasting whatever your preferred schedule; just on weekdays;

- do every other day: intermittent fasting, whatever your preferred schedule; every other day;

- do every day: intermittent fasting, whatever your preferred schedule; every single day; or

- do two meals a day: you can choose to eat only two meals a day; the best is to skip breakfast.

While you are intermittent fasting, do drink plenty of liquids. That includes water, coffee (black with stevia), green tea, black tea, seltzer water, and more. Whatever it is, it must be noncaloric and contain absolutely no artificial sweeteners.

Regarding Alzheimer's and dementia, I recommend that your intermittent fasting be at least fourteen hours, but sixteen hours is better. If you have the ApoE4 gene, the sixteen-hour range would be my recommendation.

Whatever your intermittent fasting plan, start low and work your way up. Maybe start with an eight- or ten-hour window of time between meals, and do it only three days a week. Then increase that until you get to where you want to be.

Whatever the schedule you choose, make it a habit. That will benefit your brain the most.

CHAPTER 21

STEP 5: GET A GOOD NIGHT'S SLEEP

NOT ENOUGH SLEEP is not only bothersome, making you feel groggy and irritable throughout the day, but it's bad for your health. Even worse, it's bad for your brain.

The lack of sleep has a pretty scary list of results:

- increased risk for Alzheimer's
- increased risk for dementia
- increased risk for heart disease
- increased risk for type 2 diabetes
- increased risk for depression
- weight gain
- slower healing
- accelerated aging
- fatigue
- weakened immune system

How much sleep does a person need? It varies with age, but it's safe to say that we all need seven to eight hours of sleep a night. Teens need eight to ten, but few of them get that much.[1]

The average American gets 6.8 hours of sleep a night.[2] That's close, but your body needs a consistent seven to eight hours of sleep each night.

Over the years, I've seen a lot of patients who, among other things, suffered from a lack of sleep. They always have the usual reasons for not being able to sleep (i.e., noise, work schedule, heat, TV on, lights on, medications, worry, stress, and more), but some patients had less common causes for not getting the sleep they needed.

Their causes may help you. Here are a few of them:

Can't Sleep? It May Be Your Hormones

Many years ago I had a forty-year-old patient who struggled with falling asleep, and before she even got out of bed, she said she already felt exhausted.

In looking at her blood work, I immediately noticed that her progesterone hormone level was below 0.2 ng/ml. Ideally, it should have been around 10–20 ng/ml. With progesterone levels that low, falling asleep would be very difficult.

I put her on a bioidentical micronized progesterone hormone (more about that in chapter 26), and within a couple of weeks, she was falling asleep quickly and waking refreshed. For her, it was simply her hormones out of balance.

Can't Sleep? It May Be What You Ate or Drank

I've seen many different foods cause people to lose sleep at night. For many, their body is reacting to something they ate. Maybe it's beans, spicy foods, peppers, or gluten, or it could be as simple as eating a large meal too close to bedtime. It could be most anything, so be aware and adjust. There are also many foods that trigger reflux and heartburn. They are listed in my book *Dr. Colbert's Healthy Gut Zone.*

Caffeine too close to bedtime is a common cause of a poor night's sleep. Some people need to stop drinking coffee, tea, or energy drinks by noon if they are sensitive to caffeine, but most are fine with drinking caffeinated beverages until 3 p.m. Some people can go much later. Again, be aware and adjust as needed.

Alcohol is another cause of poor sleep. It does make you drowsy, but alcohol is unique in that it keeps you from going into a deep restorative sleep. That is another reason alcohol before bed is not recommended.

Another cause of troubled sleep is artificial sweeteners. One of the known side effects of the artificial sweetener Aspartame, besides headaches, mood swings, blurry vision, memory loss, and more, is having trouble sleeping and insomnia.[3]

Besides, artificial sweeteners are known dementogens, and you don't want them in your body or brain anyway, but if you have trouble sleeping and are perhaps drinking soft drinks or eating processed foods with aspartame, that may explain insomnia or sleeping issues. As you decrease your consumption of foods with aspartame, your sleep should improve.

The best way to make sure what you eat does not keep you up at night is to eat your last meal or snack at least three hours before bed.

If you are hungry during that time but want to maintain your intermittent fasting schedule (see chapter 22), have 1 tablespoon (full to heaping) of fiber (psyllium husk powder) or Fiber Zone (see appendix F) in 4 oz of cold water. A tablespoon of psyllium husk powder has 8 grams of carbs, but it's all from fiber, so it's 0 grams of net carbs per serving.

IT'S A FACT

Coffee is a good source of antioxidants (polyphenols), but if it keeps you from sleeping or makes your heart beat irregularly, you shouldn't drink it.[4]

Can't Sleep? It May Be Sleep Apnea

Patients with sleep apnea are typically tired when they wake up, and their spouses will tell you that during the night, they were gasping for air, snoring loudly, or even not breathing for ten to thirty seconds at a time. (Those are the most common signs of sleep apnea.)

As people get older and gain weight (especially those who are obese or have a large neck—seventeen inches or more for men and sixteen inches or more for women), the chances of having sleep apnea increase.

Sleep apnea starves your brain of oxygen, which is why it's so bad for your brain and causes memory loss. This makes sense because the brain's neurons die if they don't get enough oxygen.

If you have sleep apnea or think you may have it, you need a sleep study. A simple and inexpensive pulse oximeter will tell you instantly what your oxygen levels are, and they should be 95–98 percent. Levels below 90 percent indicate low oxygen.

However, you should ideally have a sleep study. You can also do this via wrist pulse oximeter with a silicone probe to wear on your finger with an oxygen monitor that allows you to monitor and review your oxygen data. These can be purchased online for around $100.

If you have mild sleep apnea, weight loss of more than twenty pounds or a dental or nasal device can help. But if you have more severe sleep apnea, I strongly suggest you get fitted for a CPAP machine. These machines increase your oxygen levels at night, ensuring your brain is not starved of oxygen.

For many of my patients, getting a CPAP machine improved their sleep and helped them dream again, and for many, it fixed or improved their memory-related issues.

Snap Diagnostics (snapdiagnostics.com) is one company I often recommend to patients that I suspect have sleep apnea. It is a home sleep test that measures five channels of sleep data, including airflow, oximetry, heart rate, respiratory effort, and sound. Patients sleep in the comfort of their homes during the test. Their data is then analyzed by their team, and recommendations are made.

If you happen to live at a high altitude or have chronic obstructive pulmonary disease (COPD) or chronic bronchitis, you might not be getting enough oxygen during the day! Use your pulse oximeter to test your oxygen levels several times as you go about your day. You may need to use a CPAP machine at night, and during the day, you may need to find other ways to boost your oxygen levels, including exercise with oxygen therapy (EWOT).[5]

For some of my sleep apnea patients, eliminating dairy (especially cheese) dramatically improved their sleep apnea.

Your Brain Needs Its Sleep

Getting enough sleep is near the top of the list of all the steps to prevent, slow, manage, stop, or reverse Alzheimer's and dementia. It seems insignificant, too "normal," something that we ignore all the time, but it is vital.

New research about the brain is coming out that would shock most people if they knew it.

Remember how Alzheimer's and dementia patients always have amyloid plaque buildup in the hippocampus area of the brain? And how many of the dementogens increase that plaque buildup? And how bad the plaque is to the brain?

Well, believe it or not, sleep is one of the most effective ways to clear out that dreaded amyloid plaque from your brain!

While you sleep, a lot is happening in your brain:

- Processing data: The facts and experiences of your day need to be processed before they can be cataloged and stored. During restorative sleep, this processing happens.[6] Then your processing centers are ready for a new day.

- Proper storage: Sleep consolidates memories and helps your brain categorize short-term memories into long-term memories, declutter unnecessary bits of information, and store memories properly.[7] That means your memories are right where you put them, which directly helps with short-term and long-term memory.

- Self-cleaning: The brain's waste disposal system (the glymphatic system, similar to the lymphatic system) sweeps out old cells and removes toxic debris, including amyloid plaque.[8] This cleanup of your brain, especially your hippocampus, directly decreases your risk of Alzheimer's and dementia.

While the brain is in its incredibly efficient self-cleaning mode, the deeper you sleep, the better. Deep sleep speeds up the removal of the amyloid plaque by ten to twenty times! Interestingly, sleeping on your side has been found to clear the most amyloid plaque from the brain.

The lack of sleep does just the opposite and decreases your focus, memory, learning, and other skills.[9] And as you now know, the lack of sleep also increases the risk of Alzheimer's and dementia by failing to remove the amyloid plaque that builds up over time.

Simply put, get your seven to eight hours of sleep each night!

Thirteen Tips for Better Sleep

A lot of people struggle with sleeping at night. According to the American Sleep Association (ASA), 30 percent of the US population have a sleeping problem, and 10 percent have chronic insomnia.[10]

No matter how you count it, that's tens of millions of people every night!

Of the many reasons for not sleeping, here are my top thirteen tips for getting a good night's sleep:

1. Stick to a schedule. My brain struggled a lot when I worked all night on call. If your work isn't keeping you up, then simply decide when you want to go to bed and when you want to get up. Then set that schedule in cement (as much as you can). I go to bed at 10 p.m. and wake up at 6 a.m., and I keep it consistent, even on weekends.

2. Get seven to eight hours of sleep consistently. It is both the necessary amount of sleep as well as consistency that provides health benefits.

3. Make sure your bedroom is dark. Light increases your cortisol production and interferes with your melatonin production. Your body makes melatonin when it's dark, so keeping the lights on is the reverse of what your body needs.

4. Keep it cool. I recommend that your bedroom be at 69–70 degrees. That temperature seems to work best for most people.

5. Use white noise. White noise is background noise that drowns out distracting sounds that would keep you up or wake you up at night. I have a white noise machine in my bedroom but not beside my bed. There are also white noise apps for your phone and white noise videos on YouTube with completely black screens that will play for hours while you sleep.

IT'S A FACT

Women are two times more likely to suffer from insomnia than men.[11]

6. Cover small lights. Turn your alarm clock sideways, so the red letters aren't staring at you all night. I cover the small light on my white noise machine with black tape. If you have blinking lights anywhere in your bedroom, cover them or reposition them.

7. Don't exercise right before bed. Exercise boosts your cortisol and adrenaline levels, which keep you awake. So if you plan to exercise in the evenings, make sure you are finished at least three hours before bedtime.

8. Eat your starches at dinner. Of course, you don't have to eat starch at dinner, but if you are going to eat starch, I find dinner is the best time. It makes me drowsy, and I'd rather be drowsy at night than during the day.

9. Consider using blue-blocking glasses. This may be especially helpful if you watch TV or work late at night. Some recommend using blue-blocking glasses within the last three hours before bed. I prefer instead to dim my lights at night. But if blue-blocking glasses help you, then certainly do it.

10. Minimize electromagnetic field (EMF). This often includes computers, Wi-Fi, alarm systems, cell phones, and more and can really affect some people's sleep.[12] I recommend putting all electronic devices at least six feet away from your bed at night.

11. Consider aromatherapy. Many patients have had great success with essential oils, such as lavender oil, at night. It helps to relax their muscles and promote sleep. If it helps you, do it.

IT'S A FACT

Reading before bed helps you sleep. Studies find that 42 percent of those who read before bed report a better night's sleep.[13]

12. Consider a weighted blanket. Many people swear by their weighted blanket. For some, it helps them sleep.

13. Consider a special pillow and mattress. Many pillows and mattresses out there promise a good night's sleep. This is totally up to you, but if you find the secret pillow that helps you sleep, make it part of your daily routine. Get a comfortable mattress. Remember, your bed is your most important piece of furniture since you spend about 33 percent of your life in bed.

What about sleeping supplements?

That's a good question. For the most part, I don't recommend prescription sleeping pills for people traveling and (for only a few days) trying to cope with the differences between time zones. Melatonin is a great supplement for these patients.

Prescription sleeping pills are not for long-term use. I can't tell you how many people I have met who are fully addicted to their sleeping pills.

IT'S A FACT

"It is useless for you to work so hard from early morning until late at night, anxiously working for food to eat; for God gives rest to His loved ones" (Ps. 127:2, NLT).

Healthy natural supplements that help you sleep are a different thing entirely. I may have a patient combine two or more of these supplements since they work by different mechanisms.

I often recommend the following:

- magnesium threonate: 2000 milligrams at bedtime, which contains only 144 milligrams of elemental magnesium. Magnesium's sedative properties increase your melatonin, decrease your circulating cortisol, and increase your sleep quality. Magnesium Threonate in studies has been found to improve memory in older adults.[14]

- melatonin: 1–10 milligrams for adults, about an hour before bed and again in the middle of the night (if needed). Start low and go slow. I take 10 milligrams at bedtime and 10 milligrams more if I awaken during the night. But some patients need more.

- GABA. Most people are low in GABA, a neurotransmitter that has a calming effect on your body. I recommend GABA 500 milligrams one to two capsules at bedtime for women and men.

- 5HTP (5 hydroxytryptophan): This amino acid converts to serotonin and helps you sleep. I usually recommend 150–200 milligrams at bedtime. (Do not take with SSRI meds such as Prozac.)

- bioidentical micronized progesterone: Some women need this. I recommend 100–150 milligrams about an hour before bed, and some women need more.

For more information on natural sleep supplements, please refer to *The New Bible Cure for Sleep Disorders*.

Ideally, you can train your body to go to sleep and to sleep deeply without any supplements simply by winding down before bedtime, reading the Bible, or listening to calming music. But if you need supplements, start with one and add others if needed. Start low and go slow. I normally like listening to relaxing music by Tim Janis (on YouTube) before bed.

I recommend that you try these thirteen tips every night for the next month. If your sleep has improved, even a little bit, keep going.

Sleep is vital, but it is easily disturbed. Calmly but consistently work to improve your sleep.

CHAPTER 22

STEP 6: MANAGE YOUR STRESS

STRESS IS ONE of those things in life that is good for your body and brain, but only in small amounts. Temporary stress makes you sharp and gives you energy. Like caffeine, it helps you focus on whatever is required of you. Mild to moderate short-term stress enhances memory.[1]

However, chronic long-term stress has the opposite effect. When stress becomes severe, memory declines.[2]

This unrelenting type of stress is often found in people with anxiety, depression, chronic illness, PTSD, and chronic pain. I've even seen chronic stress be caused by worry, stressful jobs, bad marriages, family dynamics (sick child, child on drugs, family member in jail), the commute to work, and harmful routines.

Long-term stress is harmful to your body in many areas, causing

- belly fat,
- elevated blood sugar levels,
- higher cholesterol levels,
- hormone deficiencies,
- hormone imbalances,
- increased blood pressure,
- increased cortisol levels,
- increased risk for disease,
- weakened immune system, and
- weight gain.

But regarding your brain, long-term stress is literally like poison to the brain, bringing with it

- an increased risk of cognitive issues,[3]
- decreased memory performance,[4]
- hippocampus shrinkage,[5]
- death of neurons in the hippocampus,
- glucose absorption in the brain being inhibited (primarily in the hippocampus, where it's sorely needed), and
- damaged hippocampus function: forgetting, depression, memory loss, and more.[6]

Chronic stress keeps your body and brain in a heightened state of unrest. It's like being "on" or in emergency mode all the time. The body and brain simply can't handle the pressure over time.

Stress is such an important issue that I wrote an entire book on the subject (*Stress Less*). Many years later I still think stress is one of the biggest silent killers of today. Disease is almost always present in those with chronic stress, and with so much stress out there, it's little wonder why disease is so rampant.

IT'S A FACT

More than 90 percent of longevity is the result of your own choices: stress, sleep, exercise, food, and exposure to toxins. Less than 10 percent is genetic.[7]

How to Handle Stress

My advice for those under chronic stress is always the same: learn to cope with your stress, handle your stress, avoid more stress, and deal with/remove your stress.

Yes, it's easier said than done, but doing nothing is not an answer either. Though some stress is unavoidable, you would be surprised how many people just keep going, not evaluating or changing anything in their daily routines. That's not wise or healthy.

Truly, if you want different results, you must do something different. That especially applies to all areas of your health.

IT'S A FACT

Reading reduces stress by as much as 68 percent.[8] *It also helps lower your heart rate, lower your blood pressure, and calm your nerves.*

My recommendations for dealing with stress and maintaining your health are a mix of several practical options that have worked with many patients over the years:

- Do deep breathing exercises.
- Drink green tea without sugar. (It contains L-theanine, which is calming.)
- Exercise.
- Foster an attitude of gratitude: journal ten things you are grateful for every day.
- Get counseling if you need it.
- Get more sleep.
- Go out on a date.
- Have fun doing things you enjoy.
- Laugh every day. (Get at least ten belly laughs a day.)
- Listen to motivating podcasts.
- Listen to praise-and-worship music.
- Listen to relaxing music (such as Tim Janis on YouTube—my favorite is "Beautiful Sunrise").
- Meditate on God's Word.
- Play with your grandkids.
- Pray.
- Read or listen to good books.
- Read the Bible.
- Say no to more demands placed on you.
- Slow your day's hectic pace.

- Take a break.
- Turn off the news.
- Use essential oils.
- Walk your pet.
- Watch good clean comedy.

The truth of Proverbs 17:22 is amazingly accurate: "A merry heart does good, like medicine, but a broken spirit dries the bones."

All these recommendations may seem like insignificant little steps, but each is a step forward, which counts when it comes to lowering stress levels.

Every effort to handle stress is done on purpose. You have to choose it and make it happen. Seldom will it simply happen by itself. With stress, being proactive is usually required.

My Top Five Tips to Decrease Stress

All efforts to decrease your stress require your proactive participation. With that understanding, my top five tips to decrease stress include:

1. Laugh it out.

I've written out prescriptions for belly laughter to some of my patients. It may look like this:

> Prescription: ten belly laughs daily. Thirty to sixty minutes before bedtime, listen to Brian Regan (*I Walked on the Moon* and other clean comedy videos), Jeff Allen, Jeff Foxworthy, Jim Gaffigan, or John Pinette.

2. Burn it off.

Exercise is another proactive and very effective way to deal with stress. Numerous studies have found that physical exercise improves memory function and reduces stress because exercise causes your body to release endorphins, which are a natural antidepressant hormone.[9]

IT'S A FACT

"But the Helper, which is the Holy Spirit, whom the Father will send in My name, He will teach you all things, and bring to your remembrance all things that I said to you" (John 14:26).

3. Get in God's rhythm.

Get in God's rhythm. That means to get in His Word, pray, meditate, talk to Him, ask the Holy Spirit for guidance, and listen. I like to visualize God's Word. In my times of meditation, I visualize a scripture in my mind as it might have happened. It makes it come alive, and an active imagination is good for the brain. Every time I do this, I replay God's Word in my mind. Spending time with God brings me peace and helps decrease my stress every day.

IT'S A FACT

Don't multitask—it may slow your thinking.[10]

4. Cut back.

Is your life too busy? If so, it would be wise to cut back. These short-term decisions bring long-term benefits. For example, not long ago I cut back on my work hours. That gave me a window of time that I filled with more exercise. Adding regular exercise to my routine helps combat stress, but it also helps with my plans of lowering my risk for Alzheimer's or dementia. My short-term decision is extending my life!

5. Stop the little bad habits.

Many little bad habits can add up to a big amount of unnecessary stress. Stop or decrease your time listening or watching the news (it's always negative). Stop multitasking (focus on one thing at a time). Stop being unsure of your next step (make to-do lists). Stop creating or leaving messes behind (be organized; clean up after yourself). Stop technology from holding you captive (unplug, go outside, be free from your phone). Stop going solo (be social and include others). Stop overscheduling (time to breathe is good).

You are not a "human doing" but a "human being." Stop the excessive doing and just be still. Be still and know God!

As always, getting to the root of the problem and fixing whatever is causing stress to your body and brain is the best answer. It may take you time to do so, but you must do so.

For most people, their stressful lives are of their own doing. It's self-generated.[11]

But stress on your body and brain is simply not an option you want to live with any longer. Your memory depends on you minimizing and coping with stress. Jesus said it best in John 16:33 (NLT): "I have told you all this so that you may have peace in me. Here on earth you will have many trials and sorrows. But take heart, because I have overcome the world."

CHAPTER 23

STEP 7: MAKE EXERCISE A HABIT

When I cut back on my day's busy schedule to make room for exercise, I set myself up for success by viewing that half to one hour as a scheduled appointment that I had to keep. Maybe write it on your calendar as your "doctor's appointment" because you certainly don't want to miss those.

However you choose to do it, don't miss your exercise window. Your body and brain need exercise in a very big way.

Unfortunately most people don't stick to their exercise routines, if they even have one to begin with. Statistics reveal that 80 percent of the US population doesn't get enough exercise.[1]

I would expect the same numbers globally because we are all creatures of habit.

IT'S A FACT

Exercise is the single most important strategy to prevent and improve memory loss.[2]

As you would expect, those who need to exercise the most are not getting it. According to the CDC, more than 65 percent of the younger, more fit population (ages eighteen to twenty-four) get enough exercise, and then it's all downhill from there. Of those over sixty-five, around 40 percent are getting the exercise they need, and of those over seventy-five, around 32 percent are.[3]

The older population, which is right in the peak ages for Alzheimer's and dementia and countless sicknesses and diseases, is not getting the exercise their bodies and brains so desperately need.

Everyone knows that exercise is good. That's not a question. We all know and enjoy the benefits of exercise, including

- better insulin sensitivity,
- a better mood,
- improved sleep,
- less stress,
- a longer life,
- more energy,
- more muscle mass,
- more toxins removed,
- reduced inflammation,
- stronger bones, and
- weight loss.

IT'S A FACT

The average American only walks three to four thousand steps a day, or one and a half to two miles.[4]

For the brain, and especially regarding Alzheimer's and dementia, exercise offers many necessary benefits, such as

- decreasing the impact of dementogens on the brain,
- growing new neurons and keeping brain cells alive,[5]
- helping remove amyloid plaque from the brain,
- improved memory recall,
- increased brain-derived neurotrophic factors (BDNF),
- increased blood flow to the brain,
- increased brain volume,[6] and
- increased synaptic connections.

Some even argue that the best preventive measure against getting Alzheimer's or dementia is exercise. Others say that simply being *active* is the best defense against cognitive decline.

Clearly, exercise of any sort is good for your body and brain.

What Counts as Exercise?

Patients always have questions about exercise: "How much do I need to do? What is the best exercise for protecting the brain? What are my options? How much time do I need to exercise? Do I need to join a gym? What will this cost me?"

Some are asking for their family and friends. I've had many ask what exercises or exercise routines their parents should be doing to fight back against Alzheimer's or dementia.

If you are trying to prevent, slow, manage, stop, or reverse Alzheimer's or dementia, then I suggest the following exercise routine (which is in appendix B).

Your Exercise Routine to Prevent, Slow, Manage, Stop, or Reverse Alzheimer's and Dementia

1. Start low.

Start where you are and with what you have. Walking is a good option; you don't need a gym membership, you can work it around your schedule, and you can do it with your spouse or friends.

- Light exercise: twenty minutes, three times per week
- Medium-light exercise: twenty to thirty minutes, three to five times per week

It may not be as aerobic or muscle strengthening as other forms of exercise, but walking is good and certainly counts as being active. Using a treadmill works just as well.

This routine will probably get you three thousand steps (about 1.3–1.5 miles) in a day, which usually takes about twenty minutes, and though this is not intensive exercise, it is still enough to benefit and protect your brain. You may want to track your progress with a pedometer or Fitbit.

If you have a dog, this is a great excuse to go for a walk, and it makes exercise an easy habit to maintain. You may want to consider getting a dog, not only for the fun and companionship, but for the exercise benefits you will receive.

2. Increase slowly.

Maintain your walking, but begin to add both aerobic and strengthening exercises as well. Both are known to be good for a healthy, fit brain.[7]

For aerobic exercise, you may want to ride a bike in a park, swim laps in a pool, ride a stationary bike or recumbent bike, use an elliptical machine or a rowing machine, or one of many other effective options.

IT'S A FACT

"Or do you not know that your body is the temple of the Holy Spirit who is in you, whom you have from God, and you are not your own? For you were bought at a price; therefore glorify God in your body and in your spirit, which are God's" (1 Cor. 6:19–20).

Light to moderate weight training that tones and builds muscles is good to incorporate. That might mean free weights or a machine (at home or the gym) that does the job.

The goal at this stage is to increase, to move from walking to additional forms of exercise that burn more calories, build muscle, and benefit your body and brain to a greater degree. This would be about thirty to forty-five minutes a day, four to five times per week.

When this has become a habit, it's time to consider taking it up another notch.

3. Build up.

At this level, you may be walking four or five times a week (maybe walking your dog), getting your aerobic exercise in by whatever method you prefer, but now it's time to increase your overall exercise routine to about sixty minutes a day, five to six days a week.

Of the many options, you want to be sure to include a good portion of weight training (at home or the gym) because adding muscle is a multiplier to all your efforts. For example, it speeds up any weight loss efforts (even stationary muscles are burning energy), expedites the removal of amyloid plaque from the brain, and exponentially decreases cognitive decline.

IT'S A FACT

Following any four of five (according to Cardiff University) may reduce your risk of dementia by 60 percent:

1. *regular exercise*
2. *not smoking*
3. *an acceptable body mass index (BMI)*
4. *a high fruit and vegetable intake*
5. *a low/moderate alcohol intake*[8]

We are not talking about bodybuilding! This is still strength training, small-scale muscle building, and it's giving your body what it needs at a level you can easily maintain.

Adding a little muscle will help prevent sarcopenia (muscle loss usually due to aging), brain atrophy, and cognitive impairment.[9]

4. Go high.

With brain health and reducing the risk of Alzheimer's and dementia, you can take the approach that more is usually always better. That does not mean you need to be discouraged or feel pressured to run triathlons or marathons. Not at all. It simply means that the more you can do, the better it is for your body and brain.

If you are physically and aerobically fit, but you want to increase your physical activity, then I suggest high-intensity interval training (HIIT).

For me, this is just twelve to fifteen minutes a day, five to six days a week. I ride a recumbent bike for a couple of minutes, then one minute of max peddling at max resistance. This gets my heart rate up to around 145–155. Then I back it off to half the resistance for one minute, and my heart rate slows to around 125–135. Then one minute max peddling at max resistance. My heart rate goes back up.

Back and forth, I do this for about twelve to fifteen minutes, finishing it off with a couple of minutes at less resistance to cool down.

HIIT works the body, heart, lungs, muscles, and more, and is especially effective in helping and strengthening your brain.

There are many different ways to create your HIIT workout. Maybe you prefer running, riding a bike outside, riding a stationary or recumbent bike, using a ski machine or elliptical machine, or some other way—that's up to you. I prefer the recumbent bike because it is less pressure on my knees, but you do what you like best and what will most easily become a habit.

Aim for four to eight high-intensity periods and the same number of slow periods, with a two-minute warm-up to start and a two-minute cool-down to end.

You do need to know your maximum heart rate. Take 220 and subtract your age. Use that number as your max heart rate. With HIIT, you want to hit at 90–100 percent of your max heart rate four to eight times.

For HIIT you need to be healthy and not have heart disease. It's fast, and you get the benefits in about fifteen minutes. The American College of Sports Medicine and the American Heart Association recommend exercise testing for those at moderate risk of heart disease. They do not recommend stress testing in men less than forty-five years and women less than fifty-five years unless one or more coronary risk factors are present (other than age or gender).[10] Coronary risk factors include (1) high LDL cholesterol, (2) low HDL cholesterol, (3) high blood pressure, (4) family history of heart disease, (5) diabetes, (6) smoking, (7) being postmenopausal, for women, and (8) being older than forty-five, for men.[11]

IT'S A FACT

Cognitive decline can be avoided with simple everyday exercises, new study suggests.[12]

Exercise Multiplies Your Efforts

Exercise is unique because its benefits reach every part of your body down to the cellular level. But what's more, exercise seems to pull all the parts together.

For example, the ten dementogens are usually all minimized, reduced, or removed from your body more rapidly as a result of exercise. And the answers (steps 1–12) to combat Alzheimer's and dementia are optimized or multiplied with exercise.

For instance, your efforts to break free of insulin resistance are far more effective when you add exercise. Same with removing toxins, intermittent fasting, getting a good night's sleep, managing your stress, and more. If I were to put a number on it, I would estimate that exercise is a five to ten times multiplier of the effectiveness of any action to decrease the risk of Alzheimer's and dementia.

Exercise is beneficial to good health and helps with memory loss. You can't go wrong with adding more exercise to your day.

Your Exercise Habit

If you have a medical condition, you may want to consult your doctor first. Usually, starting low and going slow is safe for most people. It's also good practice and one of the easiest ways to establish a habit.

When it comes right down to it, when you have made exercise a habit, you are well on your way to reducing your risk of Alzheimer's and dementia.

Interestingly, making exercise a habit is a mental game. It requires effort and several weeks to establish a habit. You would think your brain, which benefits from exercise, would be quicker to accept and set the habit!

IT'S A FACT

To calculate your maximum heart rate: subtract your age from 220. Moderate exercise will be about 70 percent of that, and higher intensity exercise will be 90–100 percent.

Unfortunately it doesn't work that way. It requires effort to start and keep a habit, but this is your health and longevity we are talking about, so you have more than enough reason to press forward.

If you, like me, have one copy of the ApoE4 gene that increases the risk of Alzheimer's and dementia, then you have an extra reason to keep up the exercise habit. If you have two copies of the ApoE4 gene, exercise needs to be part of your daily routine.

Never forget, as I've said many times, no matter what your genes might be, the biggest factors determining your health and longevity are the choices you make (exercise, diet, sleep, stress, attitude, and more). Having an ApoE4 gene is no guarantee of anything.

It's never too late to start. Research has found a similarly lower mortality risk between those who have exercised all their lives and those who started in middle age (forty to sixty-one).[13]

The point is, you can (if you haven't already) start now and enjoy the benefits of exercise. Your body and brain will love you for it!

CHAPTER 24

STEP 8: BALANCE YOUR HORMONES

HORMONES HAVE A way of getting out of sync as we age, primarily due to age and hormone-disrupting chemicals that we have subjected our bodies to over a long time.

A small number of my patients' hormones are out of balance due to their genetic factors, but for the vast majority it comes down to these factors:

- age (Hormones such as estrogen, progesterone, testosterone, DHEA, pregnenolone, and growth hormone gradually decline as we age, especially after age fifty.)
- obesity (associated with low testosterone levels and higher estrogen levels in men)
- diet (Meats including red meat and poultry, dairy, and eggs all contain estrogen. Beef fat and chicken fat from the United States contain much more estrogen than lean meats. US beef contains much higher levels of estrogen than Japanese beef.[1] Soy contains plant estrogen—isoflavones—that have weak estrogenic activity.)
- lifestyle (active or sedentary)
- insulin resistance (type 2 diabetes, prediabetes, obesity)
- medications
- chronic illness or insomnia

- regular exercise
- adequate sleep
- stress
- the cumulative effect of the ten dementogens on their bodies and brains (all from part 2), especially marijuana, which can increase estrogen production and decrease testosterone levels in men
- hormone disruptors (Low testosterone and elevated estrogen levels can be caused by parabens and phthalates, which are in many personal care products, including shampoos, conditioners, moisturizers, hair care products, shaving creams, and gels. Parabens are preservatives that block bacteria and mold growth and are used as a fragrance ingredient for many personal care products and cosmetics. Phthalates work as softeners in personal care products, such as shampoos, conditioners, and cosmetics.)
- endocrine disruptors (These can also raise estrogen levels and lower thyroid function and include Bisphenol A, perchlorate—a byproduct of aerospace and weapons industries and found in drinking water in some regions of the USA, dioxins, PCBs, PBDEs—used to make flame retardants, PFAS—used to make nonstick pans, and more. See *Hormone Health Zone* for more information.)

These factors affect hormone levels, and as you can see, none of them have to do with your genes. In a way, that's good news because it means you can control things by the choices you make, rather than them being decided for you. On the other hand, your choices may not have been all that healthy, and then your body and brain pay for them later. Thankfully, your body can usually rebound when you make the necessary changes.

The even better news is that as we take care of our body and brain, the body and brain respond. Nobody dislikes that!

Your blood work with its target values (see chapter 18 under "trophic factors") will tell you a lot about your hormone levels and what you may need to work on.

I've written extensively about hormones (see my book *Dr. Colbert's Hormone Health Zone*), how to balance hormones, how to optimize them, and much more, but the focus here now is on reducing your risk of Alzheimer's and dementia. For most people (you included), simply doing what you read in these pages will go a long way in bringing your hormones into balance. And that, in turn, will help lower your risk of Alzheimer's and dementia.

Most Alzheimer's and dementia occur as we age, especially after our sex hormone levels drop precipitously. Early menopause before age forty has been linked to a 35 percent higher risk of developing dementia later in life.[2] Adding all this together means that while you work to prevent, slow, manage, stop, or reverse Alzheimer's and dementia, you are simultaneously balancing and optimizing your hormones!

Yes, that's true, for that's how the body works.

IT'S A FACT

Research shows that using Viagra (sildenafil) may reduce your risk of Alzheimer's by 70 percent![3] This is most likely due to improved blood flow to the brain.

Why Your Hormones Are Important

Your brain benefits greatly from the right hormones in the right amounts. That's why balanced hormones are so important, especially for the brain.

At the cellular level, hormones (little chemical messengers) are secreted by various glands throughout your body directly into your bloodstream. These hormones then travel to every part of your body to do their duty.

The hormones that affect your brain the most include

- testosterone (helps neurons survive and thrive),
- DHEA (helps decrease the effects of stress),

- pregnenolone (helps memory and protects neurons),
- cortisol (helps your brain focus and respond in a time of need, but too much cortisol harms neurons, especially in the hippocampus), and
- estrogen (for women, it improves the brain's nerve cell connections and helps the brain's blood flow), and yes, estrogen is also important for the male brain, but not in excessive amounts (see my book *Hormone Health Zone*).

If these hormones are depleted, blocked, or minimized, your brain and body pay a big price!

Too much cortisol: This is most often the direct result of chronic stress, and too much cortisol basically "burns out" the neurons in the brain. The area in your brain (the hippocampus) where memories are formed and cataloged for later use that needs these neurons the most is the area that is damaged the most.[4] Check your cortisol level if you feel you may suffer from chronic stress. Drawing your blood via venipuncture can raise your cortisol levels, so a salivary test may be the most accurate way to test your cortisol level. But still, your blood work will usually give you a very close number for your cortisol level.

Not enough pregnenolone: Again, chronic stress damages your brain. Pregnenolone can be used by the body to produce estrogen, testosterone, DHEA, and cortisol. However, when under a lot of stress, pregnenolone is drawn off to produce cortisol instead of producing the other brain protective hormones (testosterone, estradiol, and DHEA).[5] The resulting low pregnenolone levels cause cognitive decline (and weight gain, among other things). Chronic stress with high cortisol levels can shrink the prefrontal cortex and the hippocampus, the two main areas of the brain involved in memory and learning. Pregnenolone is made in the adrenal glands, women's ovaries, and men's testes. Pregnenolone levels decline with age.

Pregnenolone is a neurohormone and has been shown to reduce dementia risk and promote the growth and survival of neurons in the brain. Patients with Alzheimer's and dementia typically have lower pregnenolone and pregnenolone-derived neurohormone levels in the key memory-related areas of the brain.[6] Because all key steroid hormones (testosterone, estradiol, and DHEA) use pregnenolone as a precursor, elevated cortisol levels from chronic or acute stress will result in less pregnenolone being available for the production of these hormones.[7] I recommend micronized pregnenolone, which can be purchased at a health food store or online. I typically recommend 50 milligrams one to two times per day, and I monitor their pregnenolone levels.

Not enough testosterone: Both men and women have and need testosterone. Men have much more, about ten times more testosterone than women, but low testosterone levels increase the risk of Alzheimer's and dementia for everyone. Testosterone is of paramount importance because of all the benefits and protection it should provide for your brain: helping memory, preventing shrinkage of neurons, repairing neurons, improving blood flow, and decreasing your risk of Alzheimer's and dementia. But if your testosterone levels are low, then all this is most likely not happening.

IT'S A FACT

Please note that these hormone target values differ from what I provided in my book Dr Colbert's Healthy Hormone Zone. *With the knowledge I now have, I feel these are the best hormone levels for the brain. I have also lowered estrogen and raised TSH values due to the high incidence of breast cancer (1 in 8 women[8]). With all that in mind, here are my recommended hormone-level targets:*

- *estradiol 20–50pg/mL for women over fifty (some women may need higher levels) and 20–40 pg/mL for men*
- *FSH 23–50 IU/L for women over fifty*
- *progesterone 1–20 ng/mL*
- *pregnenolone 100–250 ng/dL*

- *cortisol (AM) 10–18 mcg/dL*
- *DHEA sulfate level for women 100–350 mcg/dL*
- *DHEA sulfate level for men 150–500 mcg/dL*
- *Total Testosterone Men 500–1000 ng/dL*
- *Free Testosterone Men 15–26 pg/mL*
- *Total Testosterone Women 50–150 ng/dL (and even higher to 200 ng/dL for those female patients with osteoporosis or sarcopenia)*
- *free T3 3.0–4.2 pg/mL*
- *reverse T3 <20 ng/dL*
- *TSH <2.0 mIU/L*
- *anti-TPO negative*

Not enough BDNF: brain-derived neurotrophic factor (BDNF) helps strengthen the synapses in your brain. Low levels of testosterone and estradiol hormones also lower BDNF levels, resulting in the buildup of amyloid plaque![9]

Not enough DHEA: One of the best treatments for traumatic brain injuries (i.e., concussions) is testosterone, pregnenolone, and DHEA, a steroid that protects the brain's neurons. DHEA has neuroprotective effects on the brain. Levels of DHEA fall with age, which leaves the brain vulnerable to toxic, chemical, and metabolic assaults. Chronic stress also depletes DHEA levels, and in one study, people under stress had "markedly lower levels" of DHEA than unstressed individuals.[10] I usually start most women on micronized DHEA 10 milligrams one to two times per day and men 25 milligrams once or twice daily.

Not enough estrogen: Estrogen is known to improve nerve cell connections and blood flow in the brain. It is also known to help protect against memory loss and prevent Alzheimer's.[11] Needing estrogen supplements after menopause is common, and they are good protection against Alzheimer's and dementia. Many patients need a little estrogen to raise their levels, and their brains turn on! I add the supplement DIM (from broccoli) 150 milligrams once daily to help protect a woman's breasts from developing breast cancer. Sufficient estrogen decreases the risk of Alzheimer's in women by up to 50 percent![12] Women need to have a normal mammogram before starting estrogen and need to have annual mammograms.

Men also need estradiol (estrogen). Most men after fifty have high estradiol levels due to the aromatization (or conversion) of testosterone to estrogen. I place these men on DIM, 150 milligrams one or two times a day, which is a broccoli extract that lowers estradiol levels. Generally speaking, the more belly fat a man has, the higher their estrogen level since belly fat produces estrogen and many inflammatory mediators. I have dramatically improved the memory of many men by optimizing their testosterone levels, which also usually optimized their estradiol levels since some of the testosterone is aromatized to estradiol. Refer to my book the *Hormone Health Zone* for more information.

Not enough thyroid: Thyroid is another hormone that, when balanced, can improve brain function. I've had many patients start natural desiccated thyroid hormone who then say (often a few weeks later) that their brain fog has lifted, their brains are refiring again, and their memory has improved. Nobody ever objects to turning the brain on again!

Hypothyroidism: This is associated with an increased risk of dementia. Hypothyroidism is associated with an elevated TSH level lab test; every six months that TSH is elevated, the risk of dementia increases by 12 percent.[13] Symptoms of hypothyroidism include mental sluggishness, forgetfulness, brain fog, feeling sleepy, lack of energy, and lack of concentration. Suboptimal thyroid tests can also cause these same symptoms. Many of my patients with hypothyroidism and suboptimal thyroid function also had significant brain fog, forgetfulness, lack of energy, and lack of concentration. Many experienced a total resolution of these symptoms once their thyroid function was optimized. I treat most patients with suboptimal thyroid function with natural desiccated thyroid, such as NP Thyroid. For more information, refer to my book the *Hormone Health Zone*.

If your hormone levels have been low and you are working to bring them up and balance them, I suggest you check your hormone numbers every three to six months until your hormone levels are balanced or optimized, then check them every six months. That will give you a very accurate picture of where you are and how you are progressing.

Getting DHEA, pregnenolone, testosterone, estradiol, and free T3 (thyroid) levels balanced or optimized is usually enough to help protect the brain from memory loss, high cortisol levels, and chronic stress.

The next most common hormone level to optimize is testosterone. (Everyone is different, so using your blood work results will let you know where your hormones are and what you need to work on.) Testosterone optimization can help improve memory and concentration. Numerous clinical studies in both postmenopausal women and men in andropause demonstrated improvement in learning and memory after testosterone replacement therapy.

Testosterone replacement therapy has shown a positive effect on spatial and verbal memory in Alzheimer's and dementia patients. In men, it has been shown that moderate dosing of testosterone resulted in improved memory, but not low and very high increases of testosterone.[14]

Men should get a prostate specific antigen (PSA) test before starting testosterone replacement therapy, and it should be in the normal range. A PSA of 0 to 2.5 ng/ml is considered safe, and you can begin testosterone replacement therapy. The normal range of PSA is 0 to 4 ng/ml. However, if your PSA is 2.6–4.0, you should see a urologist to have your prostate examined before starting testosterone replacement therapy. If your PSA is 4.0 or higher, you should schedule an appointment with a urologist ASAP and not start testosterone replacement therapy.

IT'S A FACT

Avoid sarcopenia and its muscle-wasting effects at all costs, for it opens the door to insulin resistance, type 2 diabetes, and obesity, which prepare the way for Alzheimer's and dementia.[15]

We can provoke neuroprotection for our brains by optimizing our testosterone, DHEA, pregnenolone, estradiol, and thyroid hormones. This also helps to protect our brains from the effects of chronic stress and high cortisol levels.

As I've mentioned, I've had many patients with memory loss who had previously been forced to quit their jobs get their jobs back. The difference? Their brains were firing again! They could go back to doing what they had done before. Their very lives were restored. I've seen this happen hundreds of times by balancing or optimizing these key hormones and adding Synapsin nose spray and a few other brain nutrients. (See chapter 28.)

If someone has Alzheimer's or dementia, regardless of what stage they might be at (mild, moderate, or severe), balancing or optimizing their hormones will usually be beneficial.

Every effort to balance your hormones will usually help strengthen your brain, and when that strengthens the synapses in your brain, you are making it more difficult for amyloid plaque to build up. That is always the goal when it comes to preventing, slowing, managing, stopping, or reversing Alzheimer's and dementia.

How to Balance Your Hormones

Hormone levels, for both men and women, typically begin to diminish around age fifty. That's normal, but no excuse, for there is much that we can do to improve our hormone levels and keep them balanced. The healthy protection from balanced hormones is an absolute must-have!

The best place to begin in your effort to balance your hormones is with an overall plan of good health. That is because balanced hormones usually mirror a balanced life.

Based on the thousands of patients I've seen over the years, I would say the best way to guarantee that your hormones remain balanced would be to

1. have an active lifestyle;
2. eat healthy (especially a healthy keto or Mediterranean diet; see part 4);
3. live a low-stress lifestyle;
4. exercise regularly;
5. correct insulin resistance;
6. get seven to eight hours of good, restful, well-oxygenated sleep;
7. take few or no medications, except Viagra, which may reduce your risk of Alzheimer's by 70 percent;

8. take nutritional supplements;
9. fix (not bandage) anything chronic in your life; and
10. avoid the ten dementogens (from part 2).

This list will help balance and may eventually *boost* many people's hormones. However, with advancing age, most people will eventually need bioidentical hormone replacement therapy.

Every effort taken to help balance your hormone levels is an equal step forward in A) many times turning off or turning down whatever is damaging your brain and B) turning on all the good things that build and restore your brain.

It's all good, and it all counts. Keep it up!

IT'S A FACT

If you have prediabetes or type 2 diabetes, that's usually a sign of low hormone levels. Men with type 2 diabetes are two times more likely to suffer from low testosterone than men without diabetes.[16]

Do I Need to Optimize My Hormones?

For most people, balancing and boosting their hormone levels is enough to get their health back on track and to prevent, slow, manage, stop, or reverse Alzheimer's and dementia.

Some people, however, will need more. They can tell because their hormone levels simply don't get high enough to get optimal results, no matter what they do. Their blood work will also show a plateau.

That's fine. Thankfully, there is an answer, and that is to optimize your hormones. That means we return your hormones to their levels when you were young (age twenty to twenty-five).

Sometimes, certain symptoms or signs of low hormone levels will not go away. This can result from age, medications, disease, chronic stress, toxicity, lack of sleep, diet, or lifestyle, but it can also signify that hormone optimization is the only way to boost it to the level you need.

At this point, the goal is to push past balanced hormones and optimize them. You can choose to optimize all your hormones or the main ones you are working on. It's up to you.

Look for a doctor who will use bioidentical hormone replacement therapy in the form of shots, creams, or pellets. There are many application options, but orally is usually not a good option for estradiol and testosterone. It's fine for DHEA, pregnenolone, and thyroid. Hormone pellets usually work best for hormone optimization.

Some patients also benefit from optimizing growth hormone levels. Insulin-like growth factor 1 (IGF-1) is a screening test for growth hormone, and my goal is to optimize the IgF-1 level to 200–250 ng/ml. I do this with a growth hormone secretagogue receptor peptide, ipamorelin, and a growth hormone-releasing hormone receptor peptide, CJC-1295. (For more information, refer to *Dr. Colbert's Hormone Health Zone.*)

Afterward, check your specific hormone levels regularly (two months after starting hormone therapy; six months thereafter) to ensure you stay in the optimized range.

The process of optimizing your hormones is not a silver bullet. You still need to eat healthy food, exercise, get your sleep, deal with stress, and more. But when you combine all these good choices and habits with optimized hormones, amazingly good things happen! I've even seen symptoms disappear and sickness and disease stop and completely reverse.

Optimize your hormones if need be, but at the very least, balance them. Your body and brain need balanced hormones to stand strong against Alzheimer's and dementia. (For more information on optimizing hormones, refer to *Dr. Colbert's Hormone Health Zone.*)

CHAPTER 25

STEP 9: FEED YOUR BODY AND BRAIN

THE GROWING NUMBER of people developing Alzheimer's and dementia these days is a scary, sobering statistic. It's a global trend reaching across every social and economic boundary with the potential to ruin lives and bankrupt families. It's horrible, and it's only getting worse.

And one of the biggest causes behind this epidemic is what we put in our mouths. It's what we eat and drink.

Someone with memory loss goes to their doctor and gets a prescription, often for Aricept. This medicine helps inhibit cholinesterase from destroying acetylcholine, a chemical that helps neurons communicate and is vital for memory and brain function.[1]

Those with Alzheimer's or dementia have less acetylcholine in the brain, so usually, the more, the better. Taking Aricept certainly helps, which is why doctors are quick to prescribe it.

However, nothing is fixed. Yes, there is a short-term benefit in memory, but nothing has changed to slow or stop the progressive loss of neurons in the brain. Things will usually only worsen over time because the person is "on medication," and psychologically, they feel better about it, but nothing has really been done to stop the downward progression toward Alzheimer's and dementia.

In my opinion, eating the right foods (along with drinking the right beverages and taking the correct brain-boosting nutrients) would be far more beneficial in the long run than any medication.

I would go so far as to say that the downward slide toward Alzheimer's and dementia can not only be slowed with the right diet; it can usually be prevented, slowed, managed, stopped, or even sometimes reversed with the right diet.

But without making changes with the right diet, the scary statistics will become our reality.

If that's not all (besides not stopping the progression of Alzheimer's or dementia at all), taking Aricept to help with memory loss comes with its own potential list of side effects:

- abnormal dreams
- constipation
- diarrhea
- dizziness
- drowsiness
- fainting
- frequent urination
- headache
- joint pain, stiffness, or swelling
- loss of appetite
- mental depression
- muscle cramps
- nausea
- pain
- trouble sleeping
- unusual bleeding or bruising
- unusual tiredness or weakness
- vomiting
- weight loss[2]

I don't think you want those potential side effects.

I don't recommend you stop taking Aricept or any other medication your doctor prescribes for dementia. But I do encourage you to talk to your doctor about following a brain-supportive diet and taking nutrients that support brain function, which I believe is more beneficial in the long run. Whether you've started taking medication or not, what you eat and drink will usually have more of a long-term impact on reducing your risk of Alzheimer's and dementia than taking any medicine.

What Is the Best Diet?

The best diet to prevent, slow, manage, stop, or reverse Alzheimer's and dementia is, without question, a healthy keto diet. The Mediterranean diet comes in second. Therefore, I recommend starting with a healthy keto diet and then shifting over later (if you want) to a Mediterranean diet.

I consider the Mediterranean diet easier to maintain than a healthy keto diet. Both are incredibly healthy options and the best diets anywhere, but I always recommend that people start with a healthy keto diet, especially if they have any symptoms of memory loss, mild cognitive impairment, or mild, moderate, or severe Alzheimer's disease.

The keto diet is a low-carb, high-fat, and moderate-protein eating plan, but many people on the keto diet are following an unhealthy version. The healthy keto diet that I recommend in this book and in my book *Beyond Keto* includes a lot of healthy fats from fatty fish, such as wild salmon, sardines, wild mackerel, wild herring, and anchovies, which are high in omega-3 fats and very low in mercury.

Let me ask you:

- Are you over age fifty?
- Do you suffer from any memory loss?
- Do you want to prevent Alzheimer's and dementia?
- Are you type 2 diabetic, prediabetic, or obese?
- Do you suffer from any chronic health conditions?
- Have you been diagnosed with Alzheimer's or dementia?
- Do you carry the ApoE4 gene?
- Are you trying to prevent, slow, manage, stop, or reverse Alzheimer's and dementia?

If you answered yes to two or more of these questions, then take some time and look carefully into a healthy keto diet. My book *Beyond Keto* goes into greater detail and is a must-read if you embark upon a keto diet. It also has the unique benefit of combining the best of keto with the best of the Mediterranean diet in one book.

After all, a healthy keto diet will do wonders for your body and brain, such as

- lowering the risk of Alzheimer's and dementia,
- speeding up the removal of amyloid plaque from the brain,
- fueling the brain,
- improving or reversing insulin resistance,
- boosting your metabolism,
- decreasing inflammation,
- slowing/stopping most chronic diseases,
- helping you lose weight,
- reducing plaque in your arteries,
- improving blood sugar levels,
- preventing memory loss,
- improving/curing acid reflux,
- rejuvenating the body,
- decreasing belly fat,
- stopping insulin spikes,
- increasing endurance levels,
- boosting energy levels,
- lowering bad cholesterol levels,
- reversing type 2 diabetes for many,
- reversing prediabetes,
- preventing/fighting cancer,
- decreasing toxins in the body,
- reversing dementia,
- reducing the risk of heart disease,
- helping arthritis pain,
- decreasing migraines,
- improving sleep,

- healing a leaky gut,
- lowering blood pressure,
- restoring a fatty liver,
- slowing the aging process,
- lowering the risk of Parkinson's disease,
- controlling appetite hormones,
- improving or curing constipation,
- enabling you to get off most of your medications,
- improving/curing PCOS,
- balancing and boosting hormone levels,
- helping keep your figure,
- decreasing bloating and gas, and
- lowering the risk of a heart attack.

Did you notice a unique pattern with these many benefits of a healthy keto diet? You are right. These benefits align with the list of things we need to do to reduce the buildup of amyloid plaque in the brain.

IT'S A FACT

Most people with memory loss are already insulin resistant. If that's you, you want a diet that will make you sensitive to insulin again. A healthy keto diet or the Mediterranean diet will do that.

These benefits match what you need to fight Alzheimer's and dementia!

There are many more reasons to be on a healthy keto diet, but the fact that such a diet prevents, slows, manages, stops, or reverses Alzheimer's and dementia is amazing.

Of course, you are the one who makes the decision and makes any diet a habit. I've had patients in the worst situations (diagnosed with cancer, chronic diseases, dementia, Alzheimer's, and more) reap amazing results when they chose to get on a healthy keto diet. It works incredibly well.

Prevention is always the best option, but sometimes we have no choice and need to fix, repair, and reverse a health condition, and thankfully the body can do just that!

With Alzheimer's and dementia, people are most often in the fixing phase, and I understand that, but I hope that someday there will be more people in the prevention phase. That is where we all need to be.

Feed Your Body, Benefit Your Brain

Feeding your body the correct foods will always benefit your brain. That's a direct and beneficial effect, but it's also the intended effect because we are in a position now as a country (and world) where we must act without delay.

Why? Because the typical Western diet is fighting against us. It's accelerating our cognitive decline![3] And unless we take steps to stop the slide, it will be too late.

You want a diet that improves your health, increases your insulin sensitivity, and gives you clear thinking. The healthy keto diet and then the Mediterranean diet do exactly that.

Unsurprisingly, Columbia University in New York found that people who stick to a Mediterranean-type diet have a lower risk of dementia and cognitive impairment.[4] And they have greater brain volume compared with those who don't.[5]

Brain expert Dale Bredesen, MD, gives a minimum list of what you want your diet to be about:

- a low-carb diet to minimize sugars, bread, white potatoes, white rice, sodas, alcohol, candy, cakes, processed foods, and more
- moderate exercise, walking, weights, or aerobic
- intermittent fasting twelve to sixteen hours at night between meals
- supplementing with MCT oil, olive oil, avocado oil, and nuts[6]

Doing just that would go a long way in stopping the downward slide of the typical Western diet. Add in healthy fat, lots of fiber, green veggies, and omega-3 fats, and you are on your way to curing much of what ails people today.

- The healthy keto diet is perfect if you want to lose weight. Many people who have tried other diets and found themselves "stuck" have had success with a healthy keto diet.
- If you want the benefits of intermittent fasting, it fits perfectly into a healthy keto diet. If you have finished your intermittent fast, morning coffee with stevia or MCT oil powder is a part of a healthy keto diet.
- If you have the ApoE4 gene, a healthy keto diet is your best option. You may already pay careful attention to your diet, but if you have the ApoE4 gene, you need to lower your saturated fat intake to 7 percent or less.
- If you want to prevent Alzheimer's and dementia, I cannot recommend a better diet than a healthy keto diet. It boosts all the good and suppresses all the bad. Your body and brain directly benefit.
- If you want to clear the amyloid plaque out of your brain and keep it from building up, add a healthy keto diet to your intermittent fasting, good sleep, and insulin sensitivity. If for no other reason, clearing out amyloid plaque is worth getting on a healthy keto diet.

IT'S A FACT

Here are ten key brain foods. (Choose organic whenever possible.)

1. *mold-free organic coffee*
2. *organic green or black tea*
3. *blueberries*

4. *80 percent or higher dark chocolate that is low in sugar and high in flavanols*
5. *sardines, wild salmon, and other high-fat, low-mercury wild fish*
6. *avocados*
7. *pastured, organic eggs*
8. *walnuts, almonds, macadamia nuts, and pistachio nuts*
9. *curry sauce full of curcumin or turmeric*
10. *kale*

A healthy keto diet also contains a lot of healthy cold-pressed oils, such as extra-virgin olive oil, avocado oil, macadamia nut oil, almond oil, and tahini, along with sesame seeds, avocados, nuts, and seeds. Organic is always best.

Less than 10 percent of your fat intake, or about 1 tablespoon or less a day, should come from saturated fats such as grass-fed butter, grass-fed ghee, coconut oil, MCT oil, and other saturated fats.

One of the biggest sources of inflammation on a keto diet comes from eating excessive dairy. Either eat less dairy or consume less-inflammatory dairy, such as feta cheese or grass-fed ghee (clarified butter). Other foods high in saturated fats that should be minimized or avoided include beef, pork, lamb, veal, hot dogs, bologna, salami, pepperoni, sausage, and bacon.

A healthy keto diet includes 4–9 cups per day of low-sugar, non-starchy veggies, such as greens (kale, collards, mustard), spinach, cabbage, broccoli, cauliflower, brussels sprouts, asparagus, onions, mushrooms, salad greens, and more.

A healthy keto diet also includes 25–35 grams of fiber a day, both soluble and insoluble fiber, from seeds, nuts, psyllium, veggies, berries, and supplements. Many of the toxins in meat and dairy are stored in the animal's fat. When you eat a lot of animal fat and fatty dairy, you also get toxins, including PCBs, dioxins, and pesticides, which accumulate in the animal's fatty tissues.

A healthy keto diet also has moderate amounts of healthy proteins, such as wild, low-mercury fish; pastured raised organic eggs, chicken, and turkey; grass-fed meats; and sheep and goat dairy.

My book *Beyond keto* provides my protocol for a healthy keto diet and includes a healthy, lower-carb, gluten-free Mediterranean diet.

At the center of a keto diet is a natural metabolic "shift" where your body goes from burning sugars to burning ketones and fats for fuel. This shift happens when your glucose levels (and glycogen and insulin) get low enough and you become insulin sensitive because you are eating so few carbs and sugars.

If you are insulin resistant, prediabetic, or diabetic, it takes longer (usually weeks) to make this metabolic shift.

While on a healthy keto diet, you burn fat in addition to burning ketones for fuel. That right there means a breakthrough for many patients because fat (especially belly fat) is what is pushing them toward Alzheimer's and dementia.

These ketones (produced in your liver) are mostly all used for fuel (more than 80 percent), and the rest are exhaled or passed in your urine.[7]

Are these ketones good for your brain? Absolutely! The fact is,

- ketones give the brain more energy than a typical glucose-derived diet can, which improves cognitive function in Alzheimer's patients;[8]
- ketones decrease Parkinson's disease symptoms by 43 percent after just one month;[9]
- ketones fuel up to 75 percent of the brain's energy needs; however, the brain still needs a small amount of glucose; and
- when someone has Alzheimer's or diabetes, the brain no longer uses glucose effectively due to insulin resistance; however, ketones can compensate for this brain fuel deficit.[10]

As patients shift from the typical Western high-sugar, high-carb diet to a healthy keto diet, some find that their blood sugar levels drop quickly enough to make them light-headed, have blurry vision, break into a sweat, or even begin to shake.

This condition is hypoglycemia, which is more bothersome than life-threatening. A small (4 oz) glass of fruit juice will usually pull you right through. I usually suggest stirring 1 teaspoon (heaping) of fruit fiber, Fiber Zone (see appendix F), or psyllium husk powder into your juice to help stabilize your blood sugar.

IT'S A FACT

Overweight? Diabetic? Prediabetic? In one study, 94 percent of overweight, diabetic patients were able to reduce or completely discontinue their use of insulin after following a keto diet.[11]

Once your body is used to eating less sugar, fewer carbs, more healthy fats, and moderate amounts of protein, your blood sugar levels won't typically go low. Your sugars will stabilize with fewer ups and downs. Insulin spikes usually caused these ups and downs, but they will be a thing of the past, and insulin resistance will improve and may eventually resolve, which is one of the hallmarks of Alzheimer's and dementia.

DR. COLBERT'S BRAIN SMOOTHIE

- *½ cup frozen organic blueberries or strawberries or other berry or mixed berries*
- *½–1 cup triple-washed organic kale*
- *¼–½ teaspoon stevia or Swerve*
- *8 ounces filtered or pure water*
- *Blend in a Nutribullet, Vitamix, or blender.*

As done with a healthy keto diet, feeding your body the right food fuels your brain.

Quite often the brain is the afterthought. It's expected to keep up and do its job. But based on national and global trends, the brain eventually cannot perform as intended. It is unable to. And this takes us right back to the recent findings that Alzheimer's and dementia are the results of a brain trying to cope in an unfriendly, toxic, starved environment.

The answer? Simply this: give your brain the fuel it needs! A healthy keto diet will do just that. And because a healthy keto or Mediterranean diet (if you choose to shift over to it) feeds your body exactly what it needs to prevent, slow, manage, stop, or reverse Alzheimer's and dementia, you now know your next step.

The next chapter goes into greater detail about fueling your brain. Plan it out, use *Beyond Keto*, and break it into parts. Most importantly, get started today.

CHAPTER 26

STEP 10: FUEL YOUR BRAIN

THE BEST, MOST important, must-have brain fuel comes from a body that is eating the right foods. When you feed your body, you fuel your brain. That is always the case and always the best option.

To keep the fuel flowing, you need to maintain a healthy diet as part of your lifestyle. It's your habit. Thankfully, healthy keto and Mediterranean diets are well suited for lifestyles and habits. They are the best foundation for a healthy body and brain that keep Alzheimer's and dementia away.

With that said, there are specific things you can do to improve your brain's performance, but they are most effective when they are added to a consistent, healthy fuel source. Nothing can replace the right diet. Your brain's fuel comes from what you eat and drink.

As you know, doctors prescribe medications that can and do provide a temporary boost to the brain, but medications do not and cannot replace a healthy diet. As always, anything less than a fix is just a bandage approach.

Once your healthy diet is in place, there are things you can do to improve memory, boost mental energy, support neural health, clean out cellular debris, and much more. All this helps protect your brain from Alzheimer's and dementia.

Twenty-Five Ways to Fuel Your Brain

So many different supplements, activities, nutrients, habits, and foods help support, strengthen, and benefit your brain that it's impossible to list them all here. The existence of such a wide variety of brain boosters shows just how susceptible the brain is to outside forces. Some of those listed here are big, and some are little, but they all combine to make an impact.

In this case, what you see listed here are all good things for your brain. On the other hand, most people are completely unaware that they are damaging their brains in so many ways and on a daily basis. Multiply the many bad influences by years and decades, and you have the Alzheimer's and dementia epidemic we face today!

But you know better. Once you are standing on the foundation of a healthy diet, here are several brain boosters that you can put into action for additional fuel for your brain.

1. Consume healthy fats.

Healthy fats help fuel your brain.[1] These include extra-virgin olive oil, avocados and avocado oil, coconut oil (in small amounts), flaxseed oil, almond butter, raw nuts (almonds, macadamia, pecans, walnuts), seeds (chia, pine, Salba, hemp), and MCT oil or powder (in moderation). These do *not* include trans fats or unhealthy oils such as soybean, corn, canola, peanut, sunflower, safflower, cottonseed, or palm kernel.[2]

2. Sharpen your focus.

You can sharpen and improve your focus with practice, sufficient sleep, exercise, caffeine, gotu kola (100–500 milligrams once or twice a day), vitamin B5 (100–200 milligrams per day), MCT oil (½ to 1 teaspoon once or twice a day), and acetyl L-Carnitine (500 milligrams twice daily).[3]

3. Increase your BDNF.

Brain-derived neurotrophic factor (BDNF) is a protein that helps your brain grow new neurons, helps existing neurons, and encourages synapse formation. Alzheimer's patients have decreased BDNF levels.[4] Exercise, raising testosterone and estradiol hormone levels, intermittent fasting, and ketones from being on a healthy keto diet will raise your BDNF levels. Also, a whole coffee fruit extract (WCFE) supplement will do it. I recommend 100–200 milligrams twice a day of WCFE. Also, 25 milligrams twice a day of tropoflavin (also known as 7, 8 dihydroxyflavone) increases BDNF, and the mushroom lion's mane increases BDNF. More on this later.

4. Protect with DHEA.

DHEA protects the neurons in your brain. Many people, especially those over fifty, may need to take DHEA to keep their brains safe. My recommendation: micronized DHEA 10 milligrams once or twice daily for women and 25 milligrams once or twice daily for men.

DR. COLBERT'S MORNING ROUTINE

I start each morning with keto coffee, which is:

- *1–2 cups of mold-free coffee*
- *½ teaspoon of MCT oil powder in each cup*
- *chocolate collagen ½–1 scoop (See appendix E.)*

5. Get more DHA.

The brain cannot make DHA but needs it for cognition, brain support, and neurotransmitters. About 90 percent of omega-3 fatty acids in the brain are DHA, and DHA is one of the main fats for synapses.[5] Look for omega-3 (fish oil) with at least a 1-to-1 ratio or more of DHA to EPA. Fish is an excellent source of DHA. Choose fish high in omega-3 but low in mercury and toxins, such as SMASH fish: sardines, mackerel, anchovies, wild salmon, and herring. Vegans and vegetarians are often woefully low in DHA, which is bad for the brain.

The truth is that most people are not getting enough DHA in their diet. How much DHA do people need? I recommend 1000 milligrams two times per day. I personally take 2000 milligrams two times per day. The FDA claims that Omega-3 supplements containing EPA and DHA are safe if doses don't exceed 3000 milligrams per day. The European Food Safety Authority says supplementing up to 5000 milligrams of EPA and DHA daily is safe.[6] If you have the ApoE4 gene, you need even more DHA. Vegans can take algal oil, which is vegan and has a very high ratio of DHA to EPA.

6. Support brain health with Synapsin.

This nasal spray is a blend of ginsenoside Rg3, nicotinamide riboside, and methylcobalamin, which is the active form of vitamin B12. It supports neurological health and cognitive health. Ask your doctor for a prescription. I prescribe this commonly for patients with any memory problem—mild, moderate, or severe. Rg3 is isolated from Panax ginseng and is neuroprotective. Nicotinamide riboside provides increased NAD+ levels for neurons, which also has neuroprotective effects and improves mitochondria metabolism in the neurons. Methylcobalamin lowers homocysteine levels.

7. Take lion's mane for better memory.

Taking lion's mane (a mushroom) has been found to help improve cognitive function and prevent deterioration, among many other health benefits.[7] This supplement is available in most health food stores. One of my patients with diabetes had a stroke and lost his memory. He started taking lion's mane 250–500 milligrams three times per day, and it helped his full memory return! Lion's mane stimulates the production of both nerve growth factor (NGF) and brain-derived neurotrophic factor (BDNF).

IT'S A FACT

The average person eating the typical Western diet living the normal sedentary lifestyle has a brain running on empty.

8. Help heal leaky gut with bone broth.

Bone broth has glutamine, an amino acid that helps heal leaky gut.[8] You can make your own bone broth. Adjust as needed, but one simple recipe includes 2 pounds of pastured animal bones in 2 quarts of water. Add salt, onions, garlic, 1 tablespoon of vinegar, and other spices. Slow-cook or pressure-cook. Drink a cup daily, freeze extra if you made a large batch, and use in meals.

9. Curb inflammation with curcumin.

Curcumin, the active ingredient in turmeric, is anti-inflammatory and an antioxidant, inhibiting free radicals.[9] It binds to amyloid plaque, which helps your body expel it, thus decreasing the buildup of amyloid plaque in your brain. Combine curcumin with black pepper, and it increases its bioavailability by 2000 percent.[10] It also helps with memory function. In one study, 90 milligrams given to random participants for eighteen months increased memory function by 28 percent for those between the ages of fifty and ninety.[11]

10. Maintain brain health with vitamin D.

Vitamin D turns on more than nine hundred genes! It helps create and maintain brain synapses.[12] Found in fatty fish (sardines and salmon), egg yolks, mushrooms, and cod liver oil, vitamin D is often referred to as "the sunshine vitamin" because exposing our skin to sunlight increases its production. You do not want to be deficient in this vitamin, for those with cognitive decline usually have low levels of vitamin D. It is readily available as a supplement.

11. Boost key hormones.

Boosting your hormones, especially pregnenolone, DHEA, testosterone, estradiol, and thyroid, has been found to support the brain in many ways.[13]

12. Lower homocysteine levels.

Ideally, your homocysteine level should be 7 or lower, but initially aim for a level less than 10. A high level contributes to osteoporosis, brain degeneration, Alzheimer's, and plaque in your arteries and is a sign of inflammation and loss of synapse-supporting nutrients.[14] Recently a patient brought in her lab work. I had ordered a homocysteine level. Her level was 14, which, according to the lab, was normal. Regardless of what the lab considered normal, I knew her homocysteine level of 14 was quite high. (A homocysteine level of 19–20 is considered extremely high and is associated with memory loss.) But unfortunately most doctors don't know this and would have thought her homocysteine level was normal.

This toxic amino acid can be lowered with the right amounts of the following: 20 milligrams per day of vitamin B6 (in its active form as pyridoxal 5'-phosphate), 1–5 milligrams per day of folic acid (in its active form as methyl tetrahydrofolate), 1 milligram per day of vitamin B12 (in its active form as methylcobalamin), and 500 milligrams twice a day of betaine (trimethyl glycine). If someone has a major MTHFR gene mutation, they will need the higher dose of methyl tetrahydrofolate.

Vegetarians often have high homocysteine levels because they do not eat meat, which contains vitamin B12. I recommend the active forms of these B vitamins. MTHFR mutation affects about 40 percent of the population and is associated with decreased folic acid metabolism and decreased methylation.[15]

These patients are also at risk of higher homocysteine levels, memory loss, and brain degeneration. If you have a MTHFR gene mutation, you are at a higher risk of memory loss. I recommend the MTHFR gene test to determine if you have a MTHFR gene mutation and check your homocysteine level. You will need Brain Zone Basic, which contains the active forms of the B vitamins and trimethylglycine. (See appendix F.)

IT'S A FACT

Five reasons to add more SMASH fish (salmon, mackerel, anchovies, sardines, herring) to your diet: SMASH fish

1. *are a source of vitamin D,*
2. *contain easy-to-digest proteins,*
3. *contain iodine,*
4. *are high in omega-3s and selenium, and*
5. *are low in mercury.*[16]

13. Heal your gut.

Without a healthy gut, it will be a very slow and difficult process (if not impossible) to prevent, slow, manage, stop, or reverse Alzheimer's and dementia. Having a healthy gut is vital! Some even call the gut the "second brain," which only shows how important the gut is.[17] A healthy gut is one of the best defenses against Alzheimer's, dementia, and Parkinson's. Simply put, you must heal your gut. That usually begins with killing any bad bacteria. Next, you must plant good bacteria. After you repair your gut, you must avoid whatever caused your gut troubles in the first place.[18] Bone broth soup daily, collagen, and other powerful probiotics will also help heal your gut. Use my *Healthy Gut Zone* book for steps, recipes, and more information.

14. Get adequate zinc.

Being deficient in zinc is common for Alzheimer's and dementia patients. Without adequate zinc, copper may build up, causing inflammation and amyloid plaque in your brain. Aim for a 1-to-1 copper-to-zinc ratio by taking zinc supplements. I suggest 15–20 milligrams of zinc per day but not more than 50 milligrams of zinc per day. Vegetarians are also often low in zinc due to their diet.

15. Increase choline.

Choline is found in egg yolks, chicken, fish, meat, and dairy. Choline is necessary for your brain because it stimulates the production of acetylcholine.[19]

Acetylcholine plays an essential role in your memory, cognition, and sleep. By prescribing Aricept, doctors are trying to raise acetylcholine levels by inhibiting the enzyme that breaks down acetylcholine. Many supplements available at health food stores will increase your acetylcholine production, including huperzine A, Bacopa, gotu kola, American ginseng, and others. DHA (from omega-3 fish oil) also increases acetylcholine.[20] Plant-based supplements are also available. I recommend alpha-GPC or citicoline 500 milligrams twice daily to increase choline and acetylcholine in the brain.

16. Up your vitamin A (retinol).

Retinol is the active form of vitamin A, and beta-carotene is the precursor of vitamin A and is referred to as provitamin A. Everyone has heard of beta-carotene, the carotenoid vitamin A found in carrots, sweet potatoes, green leafy vegetables, and more. But the retinol vitamin A (found mostly in meat, eggs, and dairy) is important due to its protection against Alzheimer's and dementia. Supplements of vitamin A retinol are available at health food stores. I recommend 900 micrograms RAE (3000 international units, IU) for men and 700 micrograms RAE (2,333 IU) for women each day. I personally take vitamin A every day. One microgram RAE is equivalent to 1 microgram retinol.

IT'S A FACT

As we age, our ability to absorb, produce, and maintain brain-friendly nutrient levels gradually declines. Supplements help fill that gap.

17. Enjoy some java.

Coffee helps you wake up; improves mood; boosts learning; aids recall; helps protect against Parkinson's, cancer, liver disease, and memory loss; and is good for your brain.[21] I recommend no more than four 8 oz cups of coffee per day with the last cup before 3 p.m. Drinking more than 32 ounces of coffee a day can increase homocysteine levels by 20 percent.[22]

18. Get your sleep.

Sleep helps your brain catalog and store information; consolidate, declutter, and store memories properly; and clear out old cells, toxic debris, and amyloid plaque. All this directly decreases your risk of Alzheimer's and dementia. I recommend seven to eight hours of sleep each night.

19. Get more active.

Exercise fuels your brain like nothing else. You don't even need to run marathons; just being active is the best defense against cognitive decline.[23] Exercise will boost blood flow to your brain, increase your synaptic connections, grow new neurons, keep brain cells alive, protect you from dementogens, improve your memory recall, boost your brain-derived neurotrophic factors (BDNF) production, and help remove amyloid plaque from your brain. I recommend at minimum walking three to five thousand steps a day (or twenty to thirty minutes of walking) five times per week. The more exercise, the better, so there is no maximum. It's all fuel for your brain.

20. Raise your nerve growth factor (NGF) levels.

NGF is a protein in your brain that boosts your mental capacity, primarily by providing support to cholinergic neurons in the brain, which are critical for forming memories.[24] In other words, NGF helps your brain grow, rewire, stretch, and learn as it did when you were young. I think of NGF as "Miracle Gro for your mind." You can raise your NGF levels by taking supplements, such as lion's mane, rosemary, zinc, acetyl-L-carnitine (ALCAR), lithium, DHEA, and vitamin D3. Lion's mane is typically dosed at 250 milligrams, and patients usually start with one capsule three times per day and increase the dose after a few weeks up to 500 milligrams three times per day if needed. On average, the dosage of lion's mane is 500–1500 milligrams a day. The dose of ALCAR that increases NGF is usually 500–1000 milligrams one to three times per day. (See appendix F for Brain Zone Advanced.)

21. Deal with stress.

Stress is a powerful force that will uproot, wear down, and eventually destroy neurons in your brain and decrease glucose uptake by brain cells, starving them of fuel. And if the stress is chronic, the process will usually accelerate. You must deal with your stress, for when you do, it unleashes a wave of healing to every part of your body. Exercise, laughter, prayer, relaxing, slowing down, and choosing to change are collectively effective ways to reduce the effects of stress in your life. See my *Stress Less* book for more practical information.

22. Take phosphatidylserine supplements.

Phosphatidylserine (often called Neuro PS or PS) is a nutrient found in many foods, such as egg yolks, organ meats, dairy, green leafy vegetables, and fish. Phosphatidylserine helps neurotransmitters, improves memory, and boosts concentration.[25] When taking PS supplements, I usually recommend 100 milligrams three times per day and choose PS from non-GMO sunflower lecithin instead of soy lecithin.

23. Consider lithium orotate supplements.

Lithium orotate promotes a positive mental outlook, supports detoxification enzymes in the brain, and boosts neurotransmitter activity and brain-derived neurotrophic factor (BDNF).[26] Lithium is not officially a micronutrient. Lithium concentrations in water and soil can vary significantly. In the 1940s doctors started using lithium in high doses for mania. Scientists have found a link between low lithium and negative effects on cognition. A large study in Denmark found that those drinking water with lower levels of lithium had higher rates of dementia.[27] With lithium, a small amount will do you. With supplements I recommend 5 milligrams of lithium orotate once or twice per day. These are available in health food stores or online. (See appendix F for Brain Zone Advanced.)

24. Increase your magnesium threonate intake.

This form of magnesium easily crosses the blood-brain barrier, improves cognitive function, protects brain cells, preserves cognitive function, and helps improve memory.[28] This supplement is available in health food stores. I recommend 2000 milligrams of magnesium threonate at bedtime each night.

25. Don't discount the power of faith!

Andrew Newberg, MD, director of the Center for Spirituality and the Mind at the University of Pennsylvania, has studied brain scans to observe the changes in the brain that occur as a result of prayer and other religious activities. He has noted that prayer activates the brain's frontal lobe, which helps protect the brain from deterioration. He also notes that the "primitive" area of the brain is deactivated by prayer, meaning anger and stress are lessened through prayer. Other studies have found that prayer boosts your immune system and helps you live longer. I encourage you to pray and read your Bible daily to strengthen your health—physically, mentally, emotionally, and spiritually.

How many people around you live on a healthy diet and fuel their brains? According to national trends and statistics, not many, if any at all. But you can and should—especially if trying to prevent, slow, manage, stop, or reverse Alzheimer's and dementia.

As you can tell, it's easy to add extra fuel to your brain. Please don't think I'm suggesting you add all these different brain fuel options to your day. That would be too much. Too much is simply too much, leading to frustration and discouragement. I recommend that you choose based on what you want, what you can afford, what fits into your day, and what makes sense for your health goals.

These are the ones I commonly recommend (specific products are listed in appendix F):

- a good multivitamin
- vitamin D3 (Your vitamin D level should be 55–80 ng/ml.)
- Balance or optimize key hormones.
- methylated B vitamins, including methyl folate 1–5 milligrams daily, methylcobalamin 1 milligram daily, vitamin B6 20 micrograms (See appendix F, Brain Zone Basic.)
- DHA 1000 milligrams twice a day to lower homocysteine levels
- curcumin 1000 milligrams twice a day
- coffee with ½ teaspoon of MCT oil powder once or twice a day

- citicoline 500 milligrams twice a day (See appendix F, Brain Zone Basic.)
- 7, 8 dihydroxyflavone 25 milligrams twice a day (See appendix F, Brain Zone Basic.)
- lithium orotate 5 milligrams twice a day (See appendix F, Brain Zone Basic.)
- lion's mane 500 milligrams two or three times per day (See appendix F, Brain Zone Basic.)

If memory is not improving, add

- Synapsin with methylcobalamin nose spray,
- Neuro Mag 3 at bedtime, and
- sildenafil 50 milligrams once a day.

The next step is to make whatever you choose a part of your daily routine. Adding these to a healthy diet makes for the most powerful defense against Alzheimer's and dementia possible. Good job!

CHAPTER 27

STEP 11: STRENGTHEN YOUR BRAIN

THE SECRET TO brain strength is consistently doing the little things that support, protect, connect, clean, grow, revive, and help the brain. Over time, this results in a healthy brain. When it comes to a healthy brain, what more could we want?

The best habits in life are lifelong healthy habits. I know people in their seventies and eighties who have maintained the same healthy habits for decades. Whether it's exercising, eating right, getting adequate sleep, living in peace, managing their stress, maintaining relationships, playing bridge, ballroom dancing, keeping a positive attitude in a negative situation, overcoming depression, or something else, they figured out how to keep up the habits they wanted.

That is the right mindset for your brain. Healthy habits have a cascading effect, where the benefits drip from one level to the next. You want that when it comes to your body and brain!

Can You Really Strengthen Your Brain?

Your brain is like a muscle. It's mostly fat (about 70 percent) but acts like a muscle in many ways. Like a muscle, your brain performs best when well exercised and worst when unexercised.

Several years ago I had a married couple in their seventies come into my office. Both were physically fit and active, but the husband used his brain regularly in his work as an architect. The wife's world was more on autopilot, where she did habitual things around the house, with friends around town, and more. Her brain was not nearly as exercised as his, and she had memory troubles.

They had a healthy foundation of diet and exercise, but she was unknowingly neglecting her brain and had done so for many years. My daily prescription for her was simple:

- read more books,
- learn to speed-read,
- listen to relaxing music, not TV,
- memorize (scripture, quotes, positive affirmations), and
- take dancing lessons together weekly or a few times per week.

Reading is one of the absolute best ways to strengthen your brain. It may help reduce mental decline in old age by as much as 32 percent.[1] Any improvement from something so easy and inexpensive is a no-brainer. Pull out your old library card or get one for the first time, buy an e-book reader, and ask friends for their book recommendations. I recommend at least thirty minutes of reading per day, but if you can raise that to one to two hours, all the better. Swap out that movie or TV show you were going to binge all weekend for a good book.

Dancing is also beneficial for both your body and brain because, in addition to exercising your body, it involves listening to music, remembering your moves, moving your body, and interacting with people—all of which stimulate your brain.

Socializing, which you can gain with the dancing lessons, is also incredibly beneficial for the brain. Like mental stimulation, social stimulation helps your brain grow neurons, regardless of age.[2]

IT'S A FACT

Monotasking or single-tasking versus multitasking: Multitasking is a distraction. It stresses your brain, gives you less focus, hurts your memory, and is addictive. Improve your focus, memory, and brain by single-tasking.

Isolation is not good. We all need friends. We all need to connect with other people. People who are married, have supportive family members, connect with friends regularly, are involved in community groups, and work have a 40 percent less risk for dementia.[3] It might surprise you that having friendships, long-term relationships, stable marriages, respect, and love can improve your brain function, but they do.[4]

If you have a social network in place, be thankful for it and do all you can to keep it. If you do not, then make it your goal to build that network around you. Socializing is simply good for your health.

Remember that married couple? The wife experienced a noticeable improvement in her memory in just a few months of following some of the protocols in this book. A year later I gave them both a clean bill of health. The point is that your brain needs to be exercised, stimulated, socialized, and pushed. That is how you strengthen your brain.

Remember the five hundred trillion connecting synapses in your brain that are constantly communicating? Well, when one brain cell sends a signal to another brain cell, the synapse between them is strengthened. The more times this happens, the stronger the bond between the cells.[5]

The constant sending of signals back and forth makes for a stronger and more-protected (from Alzheimer's and dementia) brain. But after a new task is mastered, less communication between brain cells is required. It's on autopilot.

This means that you need to continue to learn something new! Every time you learn something new, it slightly rewires and strengthens your brain.[6] This is called plasticity, and it must be something new for it to work!

They have done scans of people playing computer games for the first time with high brain activity. But after they became good at the game, the scans reveal minimal activity while playing. The brain does no more than it needs to.[7]

The new input, knowledge, or experience causes new dendrites (branches on the brain cells that grow, connect with other brain cells, and allow for more communication) to form.[8]

Your brain is growing as a direct result and not on autopilot. It is rewiring itself. It is expanding. It is getting stronger. And that is directly decreasing your risk of Alzheimer's and dementia.

Build Your "Brain Muscle"

Consider this list of brain builders to be your prescription. Feel free to share it with others and look at it regularly. Do as many as you can, add to the list, and tick them off as you accomplish them.

- ❒ Read more books.
- ❒ Enjoy the moment.
- ❒ Mediate on scripture.
- ❒ Pray for the needs of those around you.
- ❒ Learn a new language.
- ❒ Take a course on something you want to learn.
- ❒ Listen to quality podcasts.
- ❒ Start a part-time job.
- ❒ Write a book (family history, fiction, or how-to).
- ❒ Practice single-tasking.
- ❒ Listen to audiobooks while driving or walking.
- ❒ Join local groups that interest you.
- ❒ Activate your imagination.
- ❒ Self-talk. (Replace limiting beliefs with new truths.)
- ❒ Visit local museums.
- ❒ Join a writing group.
- ❒ Take a class on how to remember names.
- ❒ Learn to speed-read.
- ❒ Attend a book reading.
- ❒ Learn a song. (Sing it or play it.)
- ❒ Take cooking classes.
- ❒ Learn to juggle.

- ❒ Be part of a charitable cause.
- ❒ Master the Rubik's Cube.
- ❒ Listen to music.
- ❒ Start a new hobby.
- ❒ Journal (diary, gratitude list, prayers, ideas, and more).
- ❒ Learn to play a musical instrument.
- ❒ Use the TV for quality content only.
- ❒ Memorize scripture, poetry, quotes, and affirmations.
- ❒ Do jigsaw puzzles.
- ❒ Get a pet.
- ❒ Do crossword puzzles.
- ❒ Take dancing lessons.
- ❒ Play number puzzle games.
- ❒ Teach a class (online or in person).
- ❒ Attend a church.
- ❒ Take a self-defense class.
- ❒ Paint or learn to paint.
- ❒ Plant a garden.
- ❒ Bake or learn to bake.
- ❒ Take walks with friends.
- ❒ Plant/tend an orchard.
- ❒ Take a woodworking class.
- ❒ Learn tongue twisters to impress your grandchildren.
- ❒ Knit, sew, crochet, or quilt.
- ❒ Play board games or card games.

- ❐ Check out books from your local library.
- ❐ Be in/stay in healthy relationships.
- ❐ Know your learning style (visual, auditory, kinesthetic), and learn something new without using that style.
- ❐ Purposefully do something with the other side of your brain (left: logic, math, lists, speech, language, reading, writing; right: artistic, musical, emotions, imagination, humor).

Take this prescription seriously. Tell me if you print off this prescription (appendix D) and do almost everything on it. Maybe we can use your story in another book or on our website (drcolbert.com).

IT'S A FACT

"Let this mind be in you which was also in Christ Jesus" (Phil. 2:5).

It often takes three to six months before improvement is noticed, so keep at it. The brain is like a muscle, so you can trust that all the exercise you are putting your brain through will result in a stronger, quicker, younger brain. Trust me, it works!

None of these items are super difficult, but they are all effective at strengthening your brain. They are little steps going in the right direction.

Some of my patients have been architects, accountants, or air-traffic controllers who found they really benefit by doing things they don't normally do, such as art, music, and dance. Vice versa, it works the same.

It is the newness of each thing that helps your brain the most. Doing something you've done before is good, especially if it includes physical activity, but it's even better if it's a new experience. That will bring your brain the most benefits.

Whatever your age, your brain is strengthened by all you do to build your "brain muscle." As you would expect, the risk of developing Alzheimer's and dementia is lower in people who are intellectually active in their forties and fifties, but any effort to exercise your brain will benefit you, especially if you make it a lifelong habit.[9]

There is no age limit on strengthening, growing, and protecting the brain! The brain is an amazing creation. Naturally, the better you take care of it, the better it will treat you in return.

The Importance of Brain Training

Did you know that the hippocampus, your memory center, shrinks more than any other part of the brain? After age forty, it is estimated that the hippocampus shrinks 0.5 percent every year.[10] Of course, everyone's lifestyle, lack of sleep, environment, sugar intake, choices, stress, toxin exposure, and habits are different, but it's happening nonetheless.

The hippocampus is where it all happens. It's where the dreaded amyloid plaque builds up. But it's also where new connections form and where synapses are strengthened every time you learn.

That is the beauty of your brain. It can regrow at any time, regardless of how young or old you might be. Every time you exercise your brain, it grows. That is how you put the amazing neuroplasticity to work for you!

But for most people, their hippocampus is digressing faster than it's progressing. They are sliding downhill.

It is said that we forget about 50 percent of what we learn within one hour and 70 percent in twenty-four hours.[11] As interesting and scary as that is, it simply means that we must all adopt the mindset that we are forever students.

Always learn, always grow, and always keep looking for ways to grow and boost your brain. Like a tree, you want to be growing and producing fruit.

I like how brain expert Dr. Gary Small, says it:

> The information in our brains is passed through billions of dendrites, or extensions of brain cells, similar to branches on a tree, which grow smaller as they extend outward. Without use, our dendrites can shrink or atrophy; but when we exercise them in new and creative ways, their connections remain active as they pass new information along. And, remarkably, new dendrites can be created even after old ones die.[12]

Everything you do to strengthen your brain counts for you. Every challenge you give your brain helps keep your brain in shape.

This is especially true if you've had a setback. When the anesthesia seemed to speed up my mom's dementia after her hip surgery, my brother played the piano while she listened. She remembered the songs and would often sing along, and that helped her memory and emotions improve.

As neurons age and die, the brain atrophies. An aging brain tends to collect amyloid plaque, which directly affects memory.[13]

I've helped countless patients slow, manage, stop, or reverse their mild to moderate Alzheimer's and dementia, but time is always of the essence. The time to start is always right now.

A healthy brain is consistently learning, growing, and moving forward.

So put your brain to work! Don't overextend it but do challenge it. Keep it active. Start marking as many things on the "Build Your 'Brain Muscle'" list as possible.

Every day, strengthen your brain.

CHAPTER 28

STEP 12: PROTECT YOUR BRAIN

As we have already discussed, Alzheimer's and dementia result from a body trying to cope with its environment. Change the environment, and Alzheimer's and dementia symptoms will usually disappear.

You could say Alzheimer's and dementia are more the results of our choices than a disease. When pressed with insulin resistance from consuming excessive sugars and carbohydrates, with inflammation (from diet, infection, and other factors); starved of nutrients, hormones, and other brain-supporting molecules; and surrounded by toxic substances (metals and toxins), the brain responds as it's supposed to, and the result is Alzheimer's and dementia.[1]

Even the buildup of amyloid plaque in the hippocampus and throughout the brain is the brain's self-defense mechanism at work.[2]

To protect your brain from Alzheimer's and dementia, you must provide your body and brain with a healthy environment. And if you are trying to slow, manage, stop, or reverse Alzheimer's and dementia, the same plan of attack will work.

At all costs, protect your brain.

The best environment for your brain is one that protects it, feeds it, and grows it. It sounds as if we are talking about a garden, and in many ways, the natural laws of sowing and reaping apply.

Your To-Do List for a Healthy Brain

This short to-do list is my summation of thousands of hours of research, hundreds of doctors looking for answers, billions of dollars spent searching for a cure, and countless lives impacted. It is the best of the best, a proven way to prevent, slow, manage, stop, or reverse Alzheimer's and dementia for anyone.

- Avoid heavy metals (use chelation agents to remove them from your body):
    - mercury (in silver fillings, certain fish, certain cosmetics),
    - arsenic (in some drinking water and foods),
    - lead (in water, gasoline, paint, cigarette smoke, pipes, toys, city dust), and
    - cadmium (in certain chocolate, smoking, tobacco).

- Test to see if you are part of the 25 percent of the population that is sensitive to mold.

- Treat your body and home for mold (if needed).

- Avoid certain antihistamines long-term (Benadryl, Atarax).

- Avoid certain anticholinergic medications long-term. (Fix the problem; medications are bandages.)

- Avoid too much copper. (Take zinc supplements to maintain a 1-to-1 ratio.)

- Avoid artificial sweeteners. (Minimize sugar intake as well.)

- Decrease alcohol intake. (Dry red wine, in small amounts, is usually OK.)

- Stop drinking alcohol if you have the ApoE4 gene.

- Avoid trans fats (often in processed foods).

- Avoid unnecessary anesthesia, if possible; keep oxygen levels high, and take glutathione supplement afterward to clear it out of your body. (Local anesthesia is fine.)

- Avoid marijuana.

- Clear any chronic infections (cold sores, gingivitis, periodontal disease, chronic sinusitis, chronic bronchitis, Lyme disease, and Lyme coinfections).
- Reverse insulin resistance. (Lose weight, exercise, follow the healthy keto diet, and practice intermittent fasting.)
- Quench inflammation. (Fix it; don't patch it.)
- Restore your leaky gut.
- Do intermittent fasting regularly.
- Consistently get a good night's sleep.
- Manage your stress. (Remove stressors if you can.)
- Create an exercise habit (and stick to it).
- Balance your hormones. (Optimize if need be.)
- Feed your body the right foods (a healthy keto diet or a healthy Mediterranean diet).
- Fuel your brain daily.
- Strengthen your brain. (Every single day, exercise your brain.)

It is everything that you have read in this book. It is good for short-term results and effective for long-term planning. It is a plan, and it works. I suggest that you photocopy this list (appendix C) and tape it to the back of your pantry door. That way it's always close by and near your food choices.

In all you do, keep moving forward. Every step that becomes a habit is further protection for your brain. A protected brain is a healthy brain, and a healthy brain is your future!

CONCLUSION

I CAN'T TELL YOU how many people I've had come into my office in tears due to Alzheimer's or dementia symptoms or a diagnosis. They are mortified and often literally shaking in fear. After trying to calm them or their family members down, I explain that Alzheimer's and dementia are not diseases they caught, nor are they infectious.

That encourages them a little.

Then I explain that Alzheimer's and dementia are their brains' responses to the environment they have created. Their body is simply trying to cope.

That confuses them a bit.

Then I tell them that Alzheimer's and dementia are not the end; they are not inevitable and untreatable. The right diet, habits, exercise, and choices can prevent, slow, manage, stop, or reverse Alzheimer's and dementia if we intervene before they have severe dementia or severe Alzheimer's disease.

That gives them hope!

So whatever your reason for looking at Alzheimer's and dementia, there is hope! This may be the end of unhealthy habits, but it's not the end of your life! Armed with answers, you have what it takes. Just make sure you start today.

APPENDIX A

BLOOD TESTS TO REQUEST AND THEIR TARGET VALUES

These are most important initial blood tests for memory loss:

1. hs-CRP
2. hemoglobin A1c
3. homocysteine levels
4. ApoE gene testing
5. lipid panel
6. oxidized LDL cholesterol
7. vitamin B12 level
8. vitamin D3 level
9. DHEA-S level
10. pregnenolone level
11. estradiol level
12. total testosterone level
13. free T3 level
14. TSH
15. MTHFR gene test

The following chart is a comprehensive list of all tests you may want to ask for. It also tells you where they're available, and most importantly, the target values you will want to compare with your individual results.

Target Values for Tests Associated With Cognition

CATEGORY	TEST	LOCATION	TARGET VALUE
Inflammation	hs-CRP (high-sensitivity C-reactive protein)	Labcorp	<0.9 mg/dL
Insulin Resistance	Hemoglobin A1c percent	Labcorp	5.3 or less
	Fasting Glucose	Labcorp	70–90 mg/dL
	Fasting Insulin	Labcorp	<5.0 uIU/mL
Inflammation	Homocysteine Levels	Labcorp	≤ 7 mcmol/L
Alzheimer's	ApoE Alzheimer's Risk Testing	Labcorp	
	Omega-3 Index	Labcorp	a. ≥10 percent (ApoE4+) b. 8–10 percent (ApoE4-)
	Omega-6 to Omega-3 ratio	Labcorp	1 to 1 to 4 to 1 (Caution: <0.5 to 1 sometimes correlates with bleeding tendency.)
Cholesterol	LDL Particle Number	Labcorp	700-1200 nmol/L
	Small density LDL particle size	Labcorp	<121 mg/dL
	OxLDL (Oxidized LDL)	Labcorp	<60 ng/mL
	Total Cholesterol	Labcorp	150–200 mg/dL
	HDL	Labcorp	>50 mg/dL
	Triglycerides	Labcorp	<100 mg/dL
Minerals	RBC Magnesium	Labcorp	5.2–6.5 mg/dL
	Copper	Labcorp	90–110 mcg/dL
	Zinc	Labcorp	90–110 mcg/dL
Antioxidants	CoQ10	Labcorp	1.1–2.2 mcg/mL
	Glutathione	Labcorp	>250 mcg/mL
Vitamins	Vitamin B12	Labcorp	500–1500 pg/mL
	Vitamin D3	Labcorp	55–80 ng/mL
Genetics	MTHFR genetic test	Labcorp	If (+) with ≥ 1 mutation, need an active form of folic acid

DR. COLBERT'S HEALTHY BRAIN ZONE

CATEGORY	TEST	LOCATION	TARGET VALUE
Trophic factors (hormones)	Estradiol	Labcorp	20–50 pg/mL (Some women need higher levels.)
	FSH	Labcorp	23–50 IU/L
	Progesterone	Labcorp	1–20 ng/dL
	Pregnenolone	Labcorp	100–250 ng/dL
	Cortisol (AM)	Labcorp	10–18 mcg/dL
	DHEA-S level women	Labcorp	100–350 mcg/dL
	DHEA-S level men	Labcorp	150–500 mcg/dL
	Total Testosterone Men	Labcorp	500–1000 ng/dL
	Free Testosterone Men	Labcorp	15–26 pg/mL
	Total Testosterone Women	Labcorp	50–150 ng/dL (and even higher to 200 ng/dL for those female patients with osteoporosis or sarcopenia)
	Free T3	Labcorp	3.0–4.2 pg/mL
	Reverse T3	Labcorp	<20 ng/dL
	TSH	Labcorp	<2.0 mIU/L
	Anti-TPO	Labcorp	Negative
Toxins	Mercury	DoctorsData-Urine Metal Toxins. Optimal testing is done with urine, but serum blood testing is also available. Visit doctorsdata.com/Urine-Toxic-Metals and doctorsdata.com/Whole-Blood-Elements	a. Urine <0.8 mcg/g b. Blood <4.5 mcg/L
	Lead		a. Urine <1.1 mcg/g b. Blood <3.0 mcg/dL
	Arsenic		a. Urine <40 mcg/g b. Blood <9.0 mcg/L
	Cadmium		a. Urine <0.6 mcg/g b. Blood <1.0 mcg/L
	Benzene (optional) GPL-TOX Profile- urine	Great Plains Laboratory for optimal results. Also available from Labcorp and Quest Diagnostics.	Negative
	Toluene (optional)	Not available through Great Plains. It can be ordered through Labcorp or Quest Diagnostics.	Negative
	Glyphosate	Great Plains Laboratory	<1.0 mcg/g urinary creatinine
	C4a		<2830 ng/Ml

BLOOD TESTS TO REQUEST AND THEIR TARGET VALUES

CATEGORY	TEST	LOCATION	TARGET VALUE
Mold Toxins	Transforming Growth Factor Beta One (TGF-b1)		<2380 pg/mL
	MMP-9		85–332 ng/mL
	HLA Genotyping for Mold Susceptibility	www.survivingmold.com; Labcorp test code #167120 HLA genotyping (myhousemakesmesick.com/hlacalc)	Refer to Dr. Ritchie Shoemaker's protocol for specifics at www.survivingmold.com.
	MARCoNS Testing		Negative
	VCS Visual Contrast Sensitivity Screening	www.vcstest.com	
	MSH		35–81 pg/Ml
	ADH/osmolality		a. ADH 1.0–13.3 pg/mL b. Osmolality 280–300 mosmol
Pathogens	Antibodies to Lyme Disease: Bartonella	IGeneX laboratories	Negative
	Babesia	IGeneX laboratories	Negative
	Erlichia	IGeneX laboratories	Negative
	Antibodies to Herpes: a. HSV-1 IgM (chronic infection with reactivation of the virus may be a contributive factor to progressive brain damage characteristic of AD); IgG (dormant chronic infection is less likely)	IGeneX laboratories	Negative
	HSV-2 testing for this like above; however, HSV-2 rarely causes the progression to AD	IGeneX laboratories	Negative
	HHV-6	IGeneX laboratories	Negative

CATEGORY	TEST	LOCATION	TARGET VALUE
	VZV (Varicella Zoster Virus)	IGeneX laboratories	Negative
	EBV (Epstein-Barr Virus)	IGeneX laboratories	Negative
	CMV (Cytomegalovirus)	IGeneX laboratories	Negative
Sleep	Sleep study for nocturnal oxygen saturation		96–98 percent
Leaky gut and leaky brain	Leaky Gut Cyrex Array 2 (intestinal antigenic permeability screen)		
	Leaky Brain Cyrex Array 20 (blood-brain barrier permeability screen)		
Autoimmune testing	ANA titer and pattern		

APPENDIX B

YOUR HEALTHY BRAIN ZONE EXERCISE ROUTINE

1. Start low.

Start where you are and with what you have. I recommend starting with

- light exercise: twenty minutes, three times per week, or
- medium-light exercise: twenty to thirty minutes, three to five times per week.

Walking is a good option for starting—you don't need a gym membership, you can work it around your schedule, and you can do it with your spouse or friends. It may not be aerobic or muscle strengthening, but walking is good exercise and certainly counts as being active. Using a treadmill works just as well.

Walking for the times specified previously will get you approximately three thousand steps (about 1.3–1.5 miles) in a day, and though this is not intensive exercise, it is still enough to benefit and protect your brain. You may want to track your progress with a pedometer or Fitbit.

If you have a dog, this is a great excuse to go for a walk, and it makes exercise an easy habit to maintain. You may want to consider getting a dog, not only for the fun and companionship but for the exercise benefits you will receive.

2. Increase slowly.

Maintain your walking, but begin to add both aerobic and strengthening exercises as well. Both are known to be good for a healthy, fit brain.

For aerobic exercise, you may want to ride a bike in a park, swim laps in a pool, ride a stationary bike or recumbent bike, use an elliptical machine, rowing machine, or one of many other effective options.

Light weight training that tones and slightly builds muscles is good to incorporate. That might mean free weights or a machine (at home or the gym) that does the job.

The goal at this stage is to increase, to move up from walking to additional forms of exercise that burn more calories, build muscle, and benefit your body and brain to a greater degree. This would be about thirty to forty-five minutes daily, four to five times per week.

When this has become a habit, it's time to consider taking it up another notch.

3. Build up.

At this level, you may be walking four or five times a week (maybe walking your dog), getting your aerobic exercise in by whatever method you prefer, but now it's time to increase your overall exercise routine to about sixty minutes a day, five to six days a week.

Of the many options, you want to be sure to include a good portion of weight training (at home or the gym) because adding muscle is a multiplier to all your efforts. For example, it speeds up any weight loss efforts (even stationary muscles are burning energy), expedites the removal of amyloid plaque from the brain, exponentially decreases cognitive decline, and helps improve and may eventually reverse insulin resistance.

We are not talking about bodybuilding! This is strength training, small-scale muscle building and giving your body what it needs at a level you can easily maintain.

Adding a little muscle will help prevent sarcopenia (muscle loss usually due to aging), brain atrophy, and cognitive impairment.

4. Go high.

With brain health and reducing the risk of Alzheimer's and dementia, take the approach that more is better. That does not mean you need to be discouraged or feel pressured to run triathlons. Not at all. It simply means that the more you can do, the better it is for your body and brain.

If you are physically and aerobically fit and perhaps you want to increase your physical activity, then I suggest high-intensity interval training (HIIT).

For me, this is just twelve to fifteen minutes a day, five to six days a week. I ride a recumbent bike for a couple of minutes, then one minute of max pedaling at max resistance. This gets my heart rate up to around 145–155. Then I back it off to half the resistance for one minute. My heart rate slows to around 125–135. Then I do one minute of max pedaling at max resistance. My heart rate goes back up.

Back and forth, I do this for about twelve to fourteen minutes, finishing it off with a few minutes at less resistance to cool down.

IT'S A FACT

To calculate your maximum heart rate, subtract your age from 220. Moderate exercise will be about 70 percent of that, and higher-intensity exercise will be 90–100 percent.

HIIT works the body. I prefer the recumbent bike because it is less pressure on my knees, but if you like running, riding a bike or stationary bike, using weights, jumping, or boxing, there are many ways to use HIIT to benefit your body and brain.

Aim for four to eight high-intensity periods and the same number of slow periods, with a warm-up to start and cooldown to end.

You do need to know your maximum heart rate. Take 220 and subtract your age. Use that number as your max heart rate. With HIIT, you want to hit 90–100 percent of your maximum heart rate four to seven times.

For HIIT you need to be healthy and not have heart disease. It's fast, and you get the benefits in fifteen minutes. Consider stress testing in men forty-five and older and women fifty-five and older with one or more coronary risk factors. Please consult your doctor before doing HIIT if you are fifty or older.

APPENDIX C

YOUR TO-DO LIST FOR A HEALTHY BRAIN

- ❒ Avoid heavy metals (use chelation agents to remove them from your body):
  - ❒ mercury (in silver fillings, certain fish, certain cosmetics),
  - ❒ arsenic (in some drinking water and foods),
  - ❒ lead (in water, gasoline, paint, cigarette smoke, pipes, toys, city dust), and
  - ❒ cadmium (in chocolate, smoking, tobacco).
- ❒ Test to see if you are part of the 25 percent of the population that is sensitive to mold. (See appendix A.)
- ❒ Treat your body and home for mold (if needed).
- ❒ Avoid certain antihistamines long-term (Benadryl and Atarax).
- ❒ Avoid certain anticholinergic medications long-term. (Fix the problem; medications are bandages.)
- ❒ Avoid too much copper. (Take zinc supplements to maintain a 1-to-1 ratio.)
- ❒ Avoid artificial sweeteners. (Minimize sugar intake as well.)
- ❒ Decrease alcohol intake. (Dry red wine, in small amounts, may be OK.)

- ❒ Stop drinking alcohol if you have the ApoE4 gene.
- ❒ Avoid trans fats (often in processed foods).
- ❒ Avoid unnecessary anesthesia. (Localize, if possible; keep oxygen levels high; and take glutathione supplement after surgery to clear it out of your body.)
- ❒ Avoid marijuana.
- ❒ Eradicate any chronic infections (cold sores, gingivitis, periodontal disease, chronic sinusitis, chronic bronchitis, chronic viral diseases, chronic Lyme disease, and Lyme disease coinfections).
- ❒ Correct insulin resistance (lose weight, reverse prediabetes and type 2 diabetes)
- ❒ Quench inflammation. (Fix it; don't patch it.)
- ❒ Restore your leaky gut.
- ❒ Do intermittent fasting regularly.
- ❒ Consistently get a good night's sleep.
- ❒ Manage your stress. (Remove stressors if you can.)
- ❒ Create an exercise habit (and stick to it).
- ❒ Balance your hormones. (Optimize if need be.)
- ❒ Feed your body the right foods (a healthy keto diet or a healthy Mediterranean diet).
- ❒ Fuel your brain daily.
- ❒ Strengthen your brain. (Every single day, exercise your brain.)

APPENDIX D

YOUR PRESCRIPTION TO BUILD YOUR BRAIN MUSCLE

DO AS MANY of these as possible and tick them off as you accomplish them.

- ❒ Read more books.
- ❒ Enjoy the moment.
- ❒ Mediate on scripture.
- ❒ Pray for the needs of those around you.
- ❒ Learn a new language.
- ❒ Take a course on something you want to learn.
- ❒ Listen to quality podcasts.
- ❒ Start a part-time job.
- ❒ Write a book (family history, fiction, or how-to).
- ❒ Practice single-tasking.
- ❒ Listen to audiobooks while driving or walking.
- ❒ Join local groups that interest you.
- ❒ Activate your imagination.
- ❒ Self-talk. (Replace limiting beliefs with new truths.)
- ❒ Visit local museums.
- ❒ Join a writing group.

- ❒ Take a class on how to remember names.
- ❒ Learn to speed-read.
- ❒ Attend a book reading.
- ❒ Learn a song. (Sing it or play it.)
- ❒ Take cooking classes.
- ❒ Learn to juggle.
- ❒ Be part of a charitable cause.
- ❒ Master the Rubik's Cube.
- ❒ Listen to music.
- ❒ Start a new hobby.
- ❒ Journal (diary, gratitude list, prayers, ideas, and more).
- ❒ Learn to play a musical instrument.
- ❒ Use the TV for quality content only.
- ❒ Memorize scripture, poetry, quotes, and affirmations.
- ❒ Do jigsaw puzzles.
- ❒ Get a pet.
- ❒ Do crossword puzzles.
- ❒ Take dancing lessons.
- ❒ Play number puzzle games.
- ❒ Teach a class (online or in person).
- ❒ Attend a church.
- ❒ Take a self-defense class.
- ❒ Paint or learn to paint.
- ❒ Plant a garden.
- ❒ Bake or learn to bake.

- ❒ Take walks with friends.
- ❒ Plant/tend an orchard.
- ❒ Take a woodworking class.
- ❒ Learn tongue twisters to impress your grandchildren.
- ❒ Knit, sew, crochet, or quilt.
- ❒ Play board games or card games.
- ❒ Check out books from your local library.
- ❒ Be in/stay in healthy relationships.
- ❒ Know your learning style (visual, auditory, kinesthetic), and learn something new without using that style.
- ❒ Purposefully do something with the other side of your brain (left: logic, math, lists, speech, language, reading, writing; right: artistic, musical, emotions, imagination, humor).

It often takes three to six months before improvement is noticed, so keep at it. Build the habit, and good results will come.

If you do almost everything on this list, tell me about it. Maybe we can use your story in another book or on our website (drcolbert.com).

APPENDIX E

RECIPES THAT FUEL YOUR BRAIN

THE FOLLOWING RECIPES conform to what I call a Mediterranean-Keto diet. You can learn more about this way of eating in my book *Beyond Keto*. Recipes that need slight modification if you plan to start with a healthy keto diet before switching to Mediterranean-keto will have a "Strictly keto" tip at the end.

BREAKFASTS

Breakfast Scramble

1 teaspoon grass-fed ghee
3 tablespoons avocado oil, divided
½ cup yams, diced
¼ cup broccoli, chopped
¼ cup onions, chopped
¼ cup button mushrooms, sliced
¼ cup spinach, shredded
2 organic pasture-raised eggs
1 link cooked chicken sausage or 2–3 slices of turkey or regular bacon (nitrate/nitrite-free), diced
¼ cup berries

Heat ghee and 1 tablespoon of avocado oil over medium heat. Add the yams. Cook 3 to 4 minutes. Add veggies and cook 3 to 4 minutes more, until tender. In a small bowl, whisk eggs. Add to veggies and stir until desired doneness. Top with diced meat of your choice. Drizzle with remaining avocado oil. Serve with a side of berries. (1 serving)

Strictly keto: Women use 2 eggs, men use 3 eggs, and omit the yams and berries.

Fruit and Almond Pancakes

FRUIT SYRUP

½ cup strawberries
½ cup chopped peaches
3 tablespoons avocado oil
1 tablespoon grass-fed ghee
½ teaspoon debittered stevia (optional)

PANCAKES

4 large eggs
½ cup almond flour
1 tablespoon stevia (debittered)
¼ teaspoon baking powder
¼ cup avocado oil
¼ cup sliced or slivered almonds
Coconut cream (optional)
Organic natural almond or peanut butter (optional)

Cook strawberries, peaches, avocado oil, and ghee over low heat until fruit is soft. Stir in stevia and let cool. In a small bowl, whisk eggs. In a separate bowl, combine almond flour, stevia, and baking powder. Stir half of the avocado oil into the eggs. Whisk dry ingredients into egg mixture. Use remaining avocado oil to grease a griddle or frying pan. Heat over medium-low heat. Ladle ¼ cup of batter onto pan. Sprinkle almonds on top of each pancake. Flip pancakes after 2 to 3 minutes, when edges are no longer moist. Top with fruit syrup. If desired, add a dollop of coconut cream sweetened with stevia, or spread natural almond butter or peanut butter on pancakes before topping with syrup. Makes 6 pancakes.

Strictly keto: Omit the peaches from the syrup and use 1 cup strawberries. If you choose to top pancakes with nut butter, use almond butter instead of peanut butter. Suggested serving: 2 pancakes for women and 3 pancakes for men with 3 tablespoons syrup.

Chocolate Peanut Butter Shake

1 cup unsweetened almond or coconut milk
½–1 teaspoon dark unsweetened cocoa powder
¼–½ teaspoon stevia (debittered)

1 tablespoon avocado or macadamia nut oil (2 tablespoons for men)
2 tablespoons organic peanut butter or almond butter
1 scoop Keto Zone chocolate hydrolyzed collagen protein powder
½ cup ice

Place all the ingredients in a blender and process until smooth. (1 serving)

Strictly keto: Use almond butter.

Salmon and Avocado Lettuce Wraps

2–4 butter lettuce leaves
1 medium avocado, cut into wedges
2–4 tomato slices
2–4 onion slices
6–8 ounces smoked salmon slices (my favorite is Biltmore wild Alaskan sockeye salmon)
Lemon wedges
Himalayan salt
White or black sesame seeds

Place tomato and onion slices in bottom of each butter lettuce leaf. Layer smoked salmon on top. Add 2 avocado wedges to each wrap and mash down slightly with a fork. Sprinkle with lemon juice, salt, and sesame seeds. Suggested portion size: 6 ounces salmon for women and 8 ounces salmon for men. (1 serving)

Keto Breakfast Porridge

2 tablespoons ground flaxseed
2 tablespoons ground chia seeds
2 tablespoons unsweetened shredded coconut
1–2 teaspoons granulated sweetener of choice (erythritol, monk fruit, debittered stevia)
½ cup hot unsweetened oat, almond, or coconut milk
½–1 cup cold unsweetened oat, almond, or coconut milk
3 tablespoons chopped nuts (hazelnuts, walnuts, almonds, pecans)
¼ cup raspberries, strawberries, blueberries, or blackberries

Dash of cinnamon or nutmeg (optional)
Splash of vanilla extract (optional)

Combine dry ingredients in a small bowl. Add the hot liquid and stir well. It will be thick! Add the cold liquid, stirring until desired consistency, similar to oatmeal. Stir in nuts, berries, and spices. To prepare the night before, add an extra 4 tablespoons of liquid to thin mixture. Place it in fridge. (1 serving)

Strictly keto: Use coconut or almond milk.

Quick Berry Muffin

3 tablespoons almond flour
1 tablespoon coconut flour
1 tablespoon erythritol or ½ teaspoon stevia (debittered)
¼ teaspoon baking powder
Pinch of salt
1 large egg
1 teaspoon grass-fed ghee (melted and cooled)
2 tablespoons avocado oil (3 tablespoons for men.)
¼ teaspoon vanilla extract
8 blueberries or raspberries

Whisk the flours, sweetener, baking powder, and salt in a large microwave-safe mug. In a separate small bowl, whisk the egg, ghee, oil, and vanilla. Mix into the dry ingredients. Gently stir in the blueberries. Smooth the top of the batter. Place mug in the microwave for 1 minute 15 seconds. If the muffin is not cooked through, cook 15 seconds more. Carefully remove the hot mug from the microwave. Flip it upside down over a plate. Spread with ghee if desired. (1 serving)

Berry Power Smoothie

1 cup unsweetened almond or coconut milk, or more as needed
¼ cup frozen or fresh blueberries, raspberries, or strawberries
¼ cup clementine segments or fresh plums
2 tablespoons unsweetened cashew butter
1 tablespoon ground flaxseed or chia seeds
1 tablespoon avocado oil

1 scoop Keto Zone vanilla hydrolyzed collagen powder
1–2 teaspoons stevia (debittered) or monk fruit sweetener (optional)
Splash of vanilla extract (optional)
Dash of ground cinnamon (optional)

Place all ingredients in a blender and process until smooth and creamy, adding more almond milk as needed to achieve your desired consistency. (1 serving)

Strictly keto: Use macadamia nut butter or almond butter in place of cashew butter. Do not add clementine segments or plums.

Green Deviled Eggs

4 large hard-boiled eggs
2 tablespoons lemon juice
1–2 tablespoons extra-virgin olive oil
1 clove garlic, minced
1 red chili pepper, seeded and minced
1 avocado, chopped
Salt and pepper to taste
4 slices cooked turkey bacon or bacon, crumbled
1 tablespoon minced fresh chives

Halve eggs lengthwise. Gently scoop out the yolks and mash them with the avocado. Mix in the lemon juice, olive oil, garlic, chili pepper, salt, and pepper. Spoon the mixture back into the egg white halves. Top with bacon and chives, and serve chilled. Makes 8 deviled eggs. Suggested serving: 4 deviled eggs for women, 6 deviled eggs for men.

Hearty Vegetable Frittata

2 large eggs (3 for men)
1 tablespoon fresh chopped or ½ teaspoon dried herbs, such as rosemary, thyme, oregano, basil
Salt and pepper to taste
1 tablespoon avocado oil
1 tablespoon extra-virgin olive oil (2 tablespoons for men)
½ cup chopped fresh spinach, arugula, kale, or other leafy greens
2 ounces artichoke hearts, quartered, rinsed, drained, and dried

4 cherry tomatoes, cut in half
1 tablespoon diced black or Kalamata olives
¼ cup crumbled soft goat or feta cheese

Preheat the oven to broil on low. Whisk eggs, herbs, salt, and pepper in a small bowl. Heat avocado oil over medium heat in a small oven-safe skillet or omelet pan. Add the spinach, artichoke hearts, and cherry tomatoes, and sauté 1 to 2 minutes. Add the egg mixture and let it cook undisturbed over medium heat for 3 to 4 minutes, until bottom begins to set. Sprinkle the olives and cheese on the egg mixture. Transfer the skillet to the oven to broil for 4 to 5 minutes, or until the frittata is firm in the center and golden on top. Remove from the oven. With a spatula, loosen the frittata from the sides of the pan. Gently flip it onto a plate or platter. Drizzle with the olive oil. (1 serving)

Keto Zone Coffee

6–8 ounces brewed hot coffee
1 tsp MCT oil powder
¼–½ teaspoon stevia (debittered)
1 tablespoon macadamia nut oil (optional, for buttery, nutty flavor)
½–1 teaspoon dark unsweetened cocoa powder (optional)
1 scoop Keto Zone chocolate hydrolyzed collagen (optional)

Place all the ingredients in a blender and process until smooth and foamy. Or briskly stir the oil, stevia, and cocoa powder into hot coffee. (1 serving)

LUNCHES

Avocado and Tomato Salad

2 tablespoons extra-virgin olive oil
1 teaspoon lemon juice (or to taste)
1 clove garlic, minced
¼ cup basil, torn
1 avocado, chopped
½ cup chopped tomato
1 tablespoon walnuts or pecans, chopped

Salt and pepper to taste
1 ½ cups fresh spinach or greens

Whisk oil, lemon, and garlic. In a separate bowl, combine basil, avocado, tomato, and walnuts. Toss with oil mixture. Season with salt and pepper. If you'd like to add protein, toss in chunks of cooked fish, shrimp, chicken, or steak. Serve over greens. (1 serving)

Garlicky Shrimp and Asian Cucumbers

SHRIMP:

2 tablespoons sesame oil
1 tablespoon reduced-sodium, gluten-free soy or tamari sauce or liquid
aminos (such as Bragg's)
4 cloves garlic, minced
1 teaspoon arrowroot powder
1 tablespoon fish sauce (optional)
2 tablespoons avocado oil
1 pound wild raw shrimp, peeled and deveined, tails on
2 green onions, minced

ASIAN CUCUMBER SALAD:

2 cups sliced cucumbers
¼ cup sliced sweet onions
½ cup cooked green peas
2 tablespoons sesame oil
1 tablespoon apple cider vinegar
2 teaspoons sesame seeds
1 garlic clove, minced
Salt and pepper to taste

Whisk sesame oil, soy sauce, garlic, arrowroot, and fish sauce until smooth. Set aside. Heat avocado oil over medium heat. Add shrimp and cook for 1 to 2 minutes per side. Pour sauce over shrimp. Simmer for 5 minutes. Top with green onions. Separately mix salad ingredients together. Serve shrimp with ¼ cup of cooked white basmati rice or quinoa and 1 cup salad. (2 servings)

Strictly keto: Omit peas from side salad. Serve shrimp without rice or quinoa. To stay within optimal calorie range, women have 4 ounces of shrimp and men have 6–8 ounces of shrimp.

Chili-Spiced Salmon Over Wilted Spinach

SALMON:

3 to 6 ounces wild salmon
1 tablespoon extra-virgin olive oil
¼ teaspoon garlic powder or to taste
¼ teaspoon chili powder or to taste
Salt and pepper to taste
Juice of ½ lemon

SPINACH:

1 tablespoon grass-fed ghee
1 10-ounce bag baby spinach
1 garlic clove, minced
2 tablespoons extra-virgin olive oil
Juice of ½ lemon
Salt and pepper to taste
¼ cup gluten-free pasta (optional)

Brush salmon with olive oil. Sprinkle with garlic powder, chili powder, salt, and pepper. Grill over medium heat until fish flakes easily with fork. Remove from heat, and drizzle with lemon juice and olive oil. Heat ghee in a large skillet over low heat. Add the spinach and cook until just wilted. Add the garlic, salt, and pepper, and cook 1 minute.

Remove from heat. Drizzle with olive oil and lemon. Break up salmon into bite-size pieces. Toss with spinach and serve with ¼ cup of gluten-free garbanzo/chickpea pasta if desired. Sprinkle with extra lemon juice, olive oil, salt, and pepper as needed. (1 serving)

Strictly keto: Omit the gluten-free pasta; serve salmon over the spinach. I recommend women have 3 ounces of salmon and drizzle only 1 tablespoon of olive oil over spinach.

Seeded Bread Sandwiches

BREAD:

3 tablespoons ground chia seeds

3 tablespoons ground psyllium seeds
¾ cup raw sunflower seeds
¾ cup ground flaxseeds
1 cup ground hemp seeds
¾ cup ground pumpkin seeds
1 teaspoon salt
½ teaspoon stevia (1 packet)
1½ cups water
1½ tablespoons avocado oil
1½ tablespoons grass-fed ghee, melted

SANDWICH FILLINGS:

Nitrate-/nitrite-free ham or turkey
Avocado wedges
Sliced tomato
Sliced cucumber
Hummus
Feta cheese
Avocado oil mayonnaise
Yellow or stone-ground mustard

Combine seeds, salt, and stevia in a large bowl. In a separate bowl, whisk together the water, oil, and ghee. Pour the liquid mixture into the seed mixture. Mix well. Let stand for 2 to 3 hours. Preheat the oven to 350. Line a loaf pan with parchment paper. Pour batter into the pan, and bake 70 to 80 minutes. Cool completely, then slice for sandwiches. Makes 10 slices. (10 servings)

Build sandwiches with fillings of choice, staying mindful of your macros. Serve sandwich with a side of guacamole and a few (four or five) cassava chips.

Strictly keto: Serve guacamole with celery or jicama slices instead of cassava chips. Make sure sandwich fillings don't exceed 200 calories. Women, use 1 slice of bread and make sandwich open-faced to keep calories between 450 and 600.

Keto Burgers and Sweet Potato Wedges

2 sweet potatoes, cut into wedges
1 tablespoon avocado oil
Salt and pepper

1 pound grass-fed ground beef
2 teaspoons garlic powder
1 teaspoon salt
½ teaspoon pepper
½ cup feta cheese
Romaine or butter lettuce
Tomato slices (optional)
Onion slices (optional)
Avocado slices (optional)
Mustard (optional)
Avocado oil mayo (optional)

Preheat oven to 400. Drizzle sweet potato wedges with avocado oil and season with salt and pepper. Bake for 15 to 20 minutes. While potatoes bake, add garlic powder, salt, and pepper to ground beef. Mix well then shape into 4 patties. Grill or broil the burger to desired doneness. When you flip the burgers, top each burger with feta cheese. Serve burgers between 2 to 4 lettuce leaves, topped with tomato, onion, mustard, mayo, and avocado. (4 servings)

Strictly keto: Omit the sweet potato wedges. Instead, serve with a side salad made with 1 cup lettuce, ½ avocado, 1 tablespoon olive oil, 1 teaspoon vinegar, and lemon juice to taste or a side salad made with lettuce, tomato, cucumbers, 1 tablespoon olive oil, and 1 teaspoon vinegar. Men may add another 2 tablespoons olive oil.

Cilantro Chicken Soup

1 (3–4 pound) free-range chicken or rotisserie chicken, skin removed (or 14 ounces frozen grilled chicken fajita strips)
Organic chicken broth (enough to cover chicken, 1–2 quarts)
Himalayan salt to taste
1 cup onions, chopped
1 cup mushrooms, chopped
1 cup broccoli, chopped
¼–½ cup peppers (optional)
¼–½ cup fresh cilantro, chopped
6–8 tablespoons extra-virgin olive oil or avocado oil
½–1 cup white basmati rice, cooked

Place the chicken, enough broth to cover chicken, and salt in a slow cooker. Cook on low for 3 to 4 hours. (To save cooking time, you can also cook the chicken in a stockpot on the stove. Bring to a boil, reduce to a simmer, and cook for 1 hour 15 minutes. Then reduce heat to low.)

Remove chicken from the cooker or pot and let sit until cool enough to handle. Pull chicken from bones in bite-size pieces. Return chicken meat to cooker or pot. Add vegetables, cilantro, olive oil, and rice 15 to 30 minutes before serving so they don't get too soft. Ladle soup into bowls in 1½-cup portions. (4 servings)

For a faster soup, use a rotisserie chicken and remove skin and pull meat off bones in bite-size pieces, or use frozen grilled chicken fajita strips. Put meat in pot on stovetop with enough broth to cover the chicken. Bring to a boil, then simmer for 20 to 30 minutes. Add veggies, cilantro, olive oil, and rice, and simmer until veggies are softened. If desired, serve with a side salad made with 1 cup lettuce, 4 slices tomato, 1 tablespoon olive oil, 1 teaspoon apple cider vinegar, salt, pepper, and lemon juice to taste.

Strictly keto: Omit rice. Men add 1–2 tablespoons olive oil.

Chicken or Tongol Tuna Salad on Greens

SALAD:

3–4 tablespoons avocado oil mayo
¼ cup chopped celery
¼ cup chopped onions
3–6 ounces cooked chopped chicken or (low-mercury) tongol tuna
Celery seed, celery salt, garlic or garlic salt (optional)
Salt and pepper to taste
Any mix of butter lettuce, arugula, field greens, or spinach
¼ cup sliced cucumbers
¼ cup sliced tomatoes
½ cup white or garbanzo beans
1 tablespoon sunflower seeds
¼ cup feta or soft goat cheese, crumbled

OIL AND VINEGAR DRESSING

¼ cup apple cider vinegar
¾ cup extra-virgin olive oil or avocado oil

Onion juice to taste
Minced garlic or garlic powder to taste
Dried oregano to taste
Salt and pepper to taste

Combine mayo, celery, onion, chicken/tuna, salt, pepper, and spices. Mix well. Fill salad bowl with greens. Top with vegetables, beans, then chicken/tuna salad. Whisk dressing ingredients together, and drizzle a few tablespoons over salad. Sprinkle with feta or goat cheese. You also may substitute butter lettuce for greens and put chicken/tuna salad between 2 butter lettuce leaves and eat as a sandwich. (1 serving)

Strictly keto: Omit beans from salad recipe. I recommend 3 ounces chicken or tuna for women and 6 ounces for men.

Keto-Friendly Chili

2 pounds grass-fed ground beef
2 tablespoons avocado oil
1 medium yellow onion, chopped
3 to 4 cloves garlic, minced
1 tablespoon tomato paste
2 tablespoons chili powder
2 teaspoons ground cumin
1 can (14-ounce) diced tomatoes
⅓ cup water
1 can (14-ounce) black, pinto, or kidney beans
1 green bell pepper, diced (optional)
Sliced green onions (optional)
Sliced jalapeños (optional)
Cilantro (optional)

In a large pot, brown the ground beef. Drain the meat, reserving half of the drippings. Set aside meat. Add oil to drippings and heat pan. If desired, add bell pepper, onion, and garlic, and cook until lightly browned. Stir in tomato paste, chili powder, and cumin. Cook for 1 minute. Add water, tomatoes, and ground beef. Stir to combine. Bring to boil, then lower heat to a gentle simmer and cook for 1 to 2 hours. (Alternatively: After browning meat, transfer to a slow cooker and add remaining ingredients, except beans and toppings. Cook 4 to 6 hours.) Add beans and warm through.

Top with green onions, jalapeños, and cilantro as desired. (6 servings)

Strictly keto: Omit beans. I recommend men add 1 or 2 tablespoons avocado oil or a green salad with tomatoes, onions, and Oil and Vinegar Dressing to increase calories.

Fajita Skewers

1 pound grass-fed steak, cut in cubes
1 tablespoon chili powder
1½ teaspoons paprika
1 teaspoon ground cumin
½ teaspoon garlic powder
½ teaspoon salt
¼ cup avocado oil
Juice of 2 limes
1 large onion
1 green or red bell pepper
15–20 mushrooms
6 skewers

Place the cubed steak in a large container and set aside. Cut onion and pepper into 1-inch chunks. Add onion, pepper, and mushrooms to container with steak. In a small bowl, combine the spices, salt, oil and lime juice. Whisk well, and pour into the container with steak and veggies. Place lid on container, and gently shake to distribute marinade. Place in the refrigerator for 30 to 45 minutes, shaking container 2 times while marinating. Preheat a grill to medium-high heat. Thread roughly 3 ounces of steak, along with peppers, onions, and mushrooms onto the skewers. Grill the kabobs for 7 to 10 minutes, turning halfway, until desired doneness on steak. Makes 6 skewers. May eat with a salad made with 1 cup of romaine lettuce, ¼ cup each of tomatoes, onions, and cucumbers, and a simple dressing made with 2 tablespoons of extra-virgin olive oil and 2 teaspoons of vinegar.

Strictly keto: Omit one vegetable to reduce carbs. Suggested serving: 2 skewers for women and 3 for men.

Keto Cobb Salad

3 cups mixed greens
3–6 ounces cooked pasture-raised chicken or turkey
1 slice cooked bacon or turkey bacon, diced

1 large egg, hard-boiled and sliced
4 grape tomatoes, halved
½ avocado, sliced or cubed
¼ cup sliced mushrooms
2 tablespoons low-carb ranch dressing (made with avocado or extra-virgin olive oil such as Primal Kitchen's ranch dressing)
¼ cup soft goat or feta cheese crumbles (optional)

Place greens in a large bowl. Add bacon, egg, tomatoes, avocado, onion, and mushrooms. Top with dressing and cheese. (1 serving)

DINNERS

Asian Stir Fry

1½ tablespoons avocado oil
1½ tablespoons sesame seed oil
3–6 ounces chicken cut into bite-size pieces
2 cups veggies (broccoli, cabbage, bok choy, green onion, peppers, mushrooms)
1 garlic clove, minced
½ tablespoon fresh ginger, minced
1 teaspoon organic soy sauce (gluten-free, non-GMO) or tamari sauce
Chili garlic sauce to taste
Sesame seeds
1 green onion, minced
¼ cup cooked basmati rice

Heat the avocado and sesame seed oils in a large skillet over medium heat. Add the chicken, turning after 3 to 4 minutes. Cook until almost done. Add vegetables, garlic, and ginger and cook until tender-crisp, stirring occasionally. Remove from heat. Drizzle with avocado oil and gluten-free soy sauce. Dot with chili garlic sauce for spiciness. Sprinkle with sesame seeds and green onion. (1 serving)

Strictly keto: Omit rice. Women use 3 ounces of chicken and 1 tablespoon each of the sesame seed and avocado oils to stay within their calorie limits. Men use 6 ounces of chicken.

Shrimp Scampi

1 tablespoon grass-fed ghee
4 tablespoons avocado oil, divided
4–8 ounces raw wild shrimp, peeled
1 clove garlic, minced
Juice of ½ lemon
2 tablespoons dry white wine
Salt and pepper to taste
1–2 cups asparagus or broccoli

Heat the ghee and 3 tablespoons avocado oil in a skillet over medium heat. When melted, add the shrimp. Turn shrimp once, and cook until pink throughout, about 3 minutes. Add the garlic, lemon, wine, salt, and pepper. Cook 1 minute. Remove from pan. Heat remaining oil. Sauté asparagus or broccoli for 3 to 4 minutes. Season with salt and pepper. (1 serving)

Strictly keto: Omit wine from sauce and use no more than 1½ cups of veggies. Women use 4 ounces of shrimp and cook it in 1 tablespoon of ghee and 2 tablespoons of avocado oil. Men use 8 ounces of shrimp and cook it in 1 tablespoon of ghee and 3 tablespoons of avocado oil.

Mediterranean-Keto Pizza

CRUST:

¼ cup coconut flour, sifted
¼ teaspoon salt
½ teaspoon herbs and spices (any mixture of basil, thyme, garlic
powder, oregano, red pepper flakes, etc.)
2 tablespoons ground psyllium husks
1 tablespoon avocado or extra-virgin olive oil
1 cup warm water (not boiling)

SAUCE:

1/2 cup low-sugar tomato sauce
1 teaspoon herbs and spices (basil, thyme, garlic powder, oregano, red pepper flakes)
1 tablespoon extra-virgin olive oil

TOPPINGS:

Olives
Nitrate/nitrite-free sliced ham or cooked chicken strips
Artichoke hearts
Roasted red peppers
Mushrooms
Onions
½ cup goat cheese or feta crumbles or part-skim mozzarella cheese
¼ cup pine nuts, toasted
Fresh herbs (basil, oregano, thyme)

Preheat the oven to 400. Line a large baking sheet with parchment paper. In a large mixing bowl, combine coconut flour, salt, herbs/spices, psyllium husks, oil, and water. Mix well then knead the dough for 2 to 3 minutes. The batter may seem a little wet, but that's OK. Set dough aside for 15 minutes. Meanwhile, combine tomato sauce, herbs/spices, and 1 tablespoon olive oil. Sprinkle coconut or almond flour on counter or rolling sheet. Roll the dough out to ½-inch thickness. Place on baking sheet. Top crust with tomato sauce and toppings of choice. Bake for 12 to 15 minutes, or until the edges of the crust are slightly brown. Garnish with toasted pine nuts and fresh herbs. (2 servings)

Strictly keto: Omit pine nuts and use smaller amounts of the veggies. If desired, add a green side salad made with 1 cup lettuce, ½ avocado, 1 tablespoon olive oil, 1 teaspoon vinegar, and lemon juice to taste or with spinach, goat or feta cheese, 1 tablespoon olive oil, and 1 teaspoon vinegar. Men add 1 more ounce feta or goat cheese and/or 1–2 tablespoons olive oil if needed to increase calories.

Tip: This pizza has a few extra carbs, so lower the carbs on your other meals to account for them. If you don't want to make your own pizza crust, buy a low-carb cauliflower-crust pizza. There are several brands that are very low in net carbs. For instance, the Cali'flour brand's traditional flavor has 90 calories and 1 gram of net carbs per serving. (If you have a hard time digesting cauliflower, take an alpha-galactosidase enzyme product such as Beano before you eat to prevent stomach upset.) I like to put olive oil on the crust, then pizza sauce, then goat or part-skim mozzarella cheese. Then I add toppings: lots of mushrooms and onions, a small amount of ham, then a little minced garlic on top. That makes a delicious pizza!

Chinese Chicken Strips

⅓ cup quinoa
1 cup coconut milk
1 cup water
Cilantro to taste
Green onions, sliced
4 tablespoons organic gluten-free soy sauce (non-GMO)
4 tablespoons rice vinegar
1/2 teaspoon sesame oil
1 teaspoon red pepper flakes
4 tablespoons chicken broth
½ teaspoon ground ginger
½ teaspoon onion powder
6 boneless skinless chicken breasts, cut into strips
2 eggs
1 cup almond flour
3 tablespoons avocado oil

Cook quinoa according to package instructions, using coconut milk for half of the liquid and water for the remaining half. When quinoa is ready, stir in cilantro and green onions. Serve in ¼-cup portions. To prepare the meat, whisk soy, vinegar, ½ teaspoon of sesame oil, red pepper flakes, chicken broth, ginger, and onion powder in a bowl. Add chicken and marinate for 30 minutes up to 2 hours. In a separate bowl, whisk the eggs. Pour the almond flour onto a shallow plate. Drain marinade. Dip chicken pieces into the almond flour, coating all sides, and then dip it into the egg mixture. Heat avocado oil in large pan over medium heat. Cook chicken for 7 to 8 minutes, turning strips halfway, until brown and cooked through. Garnish with green onions. Serve with quinoa and a side of sautéed vegetables such as cabbage or broccoli. (4–6 servings)

Strictly keto: Omit quinoa. Increase amount of sautéed vegetables on the side to 1 cup. Suggested serving: 4 ounces chicken for women and 6 ounces for men.

Curried Shrimp and Broccoli

1 tablespoon avocado oil
1 tablespoon extra-virgin coconut oil
1 pound raw wild shrimp, peeled
1 tablespoon yellow curry powder
¼ teaspoon cinnamon
Salt and pepper to taste
2 oranges, seeded and quartered
½ cup snap peas, cut in half
Fresh cilantro
1 tablespoon extra-virgin olive oil
2 cups broccoli, chopped
Salt and pepper to taste
Lemon wedges

Heat avocado and coconut oils in a skillet over medium heat. Add shrimp and cook for about 2 minutes per side. Add curry powder, cinnamon, salt, pepper, orange pieces, and peas, stirring well. Cook until shrimp are pink and start to curl and oranges are browned. Garnish with fresh cilantro before serving.

In a separate pan, heat olive oil and cook broccoli until tender, stirring occasionally. Season with salt, pepper, and lemon juice. (2 servings)

Strictly keto: Omit snap peas and oranges. Add 1 cup cabbage sautéed in 1 tablespoon olive oil. Men can cook 2 cups veggies in 2 tablespoons olive oil.

Stuffed Pork Chops

1 slice cooked bacon, diced
½ cup chopped white mushrooms
2 ounces goat cheese, crumbled
1 teaspoon chopped fresh rosemary
1 large clove garlic, minced
2 (12-ounce) bone-in pork chops (about 1 inch thick)
½ teaspoon salt
¼ teaspoon pepper
¼ teaspoon garlic powder
1 tablespoon avocado oil

Preheat the oven to 350. In a small bowl mix bacon, mushrooms, goat cheese, rosemary, and garlic. Cut a large slit in the side of each pork chop. Do not cut all the way through. Stuff the pork chops with the mushroom filling, then press closed and secure with toothpicks or twine. Season the chops with salt, pepper, and garlic. Heat the avocado oil in an oven-safe pan over medium-high heat. Sear each side of the pork chops, about 2 to 3 minutes per side. Transfer the pan to the oven and bake for 25 to 30 minutes. Internal meat temperature should reach 145. Allow the pork chops to rest for 3 to 5 minutes before serving. Serve with ½ cup roasted yams and a side salad made with lettuce, tomato, cucumbers, 1 tablespoon olive oil, and 1 teaspoon vinegar. (2 servings)

Strictly Keto: Suggested serving: 8 ounces of pork for women and 12 ounces for men. Omit yams. Serve with a salad made with 2 cups lettuce, ½ cup tomatoes, ½ cup cucumbers, 2 tablespoons olive oil, and 2 teaspoons vinegar and/or 1 cup green beans sautéed in 2 tablespoons olive oil. Men may add 1–2 tablespoons olive oil if needed to increase calories.

Garlic Steak and Cauliflower Rice

2 grass-fed rib eye steaks, 3 ounces each
1 tablespoon grass-fed ghee, divided
1 tablespoon avocado oil, divided
2 cloves garlic, minced
1 medium head cauliflower
2 tablespoons extra-virgin olive oil
1 clove garlic, minced
Salt and pepper

Grill or pan sear rib eyes over medium heat until desired doneness. In a small pan, melt the ghee; then add the garlic and avocado oil. Cook for 1 minute. Drizzle ghee and avocado oil over top of steaks. Core the cauliflower and chop coarsely. Pulse cauliflower in food processor until it looks like large pieces of rice. In a large skillet over medium heat, heat the olive oil. Add the garlic and sauté for 1 minute. Add the riced cauliflower and cook for about 10 minutes or until the cauliflower rice is tender. Season with salt and pepper. (2 servings)

Strictly keto: Limit cauliflower rice to 1 cup. Add green salad made with 1 cup lettuce, ½ avocado, 1 tablespoon olive oil, 1 teaspoon vinegar, and lemon juice to taste. Suggested serving: 4 ounces steak for women and 6 ounces for men.

Macadamia Nut–Crusted Wild Tilapia

2 (4-ounce) wild tilapia fillets
½ cup unsalted macadamia nuts
1 tablespoon chopped fresh parsley
1 tablespoon fresh lemon juice
2 tablespoons avocado oil
¼ teaspoon garlic powder
Salt and pepper to taste
2 tablespoons olive oil
Lemon wedges, for serving

Preheat the oven to 400. Line a rimmed baking sheet with parchment paper. Place the nuts, parsley, and lemon juice in a food processor and pulse until the mixture is combined and looks like crumbs. Spread mixture onto a plate. Brush each fillet with avocado oil. Then press both sides of the fish into the nut mixture. Sprinkle with garlic, salt, and pepper. Bake for 10 to 15 minutes, until the top is crisp and slightly golden brown. Squeeze lemon over the top before serving. Serve with a side salad, cauliflower rice, or sautéed bok choy. (2 servings)

Serve with cauliflower rice, sautéed bok choy, a side salad made with 1 cup lettuce, ½ avocado, 1 tablespoon olive oil, 1 teaspoon vinegar, and lemon juice to taste or with lettuce, tomato, cucumbers, 1 tablespoon olive oil, and 1 teaspoon vinegar.

Zoodles

2 to 3 medium zucchinis
1 tablespoon grass-fed ghee
3 tablespoons extra-virgin olive oil
1 small clove garlic, pressed
Italian herbs (optional)
Salt and pepper

Rinse the zucchini and cut off both ends. Push the zucchini through a spiral slicer (spiralizer). Heat ghee and oil in a large skillet over medium heat. Add garlic and cook for 1 minute. Add the zucchini noodles and Italian herbs. Toss to coat in the garlic butter. Cook for 1 to 5 minutes to desired doneness. Season with salt and pepper. Serve with protein of choice or as a side to any dish. (2 servings)

Red Curry Chicken

2 tablespoons avocado oil
1 pound boneless, skinless chicken thighs
1 green bell pepper, sliced
1 red bell pepper, sliced
1 cup snap peas, sliced in half
1 can (14-ounce) coconut milk
1 tablespoon fish sauce (optional)
2 tablespoons red curry paste
Salt and pepper to taste
Red pepper flakes (optional)
8–10 fresh basil leaves, sliced

Heat the oil in a large skillet over medium heat. Add the chicken. Cook for 3 to 4 minutes per side. Remove chicken and set aside. Add bell peppers and snap peas to pan. Cook until the peppers are tender. Remove from the pan and set aside. In the same skillet, combine the coconut milk, fish sauce, and curry paste. Stir well to combine and simmer for 4 to 5 minutes. Chop the chicken into bite-sized pieces. Add chicken, peppers, peas, and basil leaves to pan. Stir and simmer for 3 to 4 minutes. Season with salt, pepper, and chili flakes. Serve over cauliflower rice if desired. (3 servings)

Strictly keto: Omit snap peas. Add broccoli or mushrooms instead. Suggested serving: 4 ounces chicken for women and 6 ounces chicken for men.

APPENDIX F

SUPPLEMENTS TO FUEL YOUR BODY AND BRAIN

THE FOLLOWING SUPPLEMENTS are beneficial for your brain health.

Divine Health Supplements

Available at shop.drcolbert.com or by calling (407) 732-6952

1. MCT oil powder is made of healthy fats that help support a healthy heart and brain. MCT oil also helps the liver produce ketone bodies, which put the body into ketosis and set the body up to burn fat. Take about ½ teaspoon to 1 teaspoon of MCT oil powder in coffee or mix with any hot liquid to avoid clumping. Flavors include coconut cream, hazelnut, French vanilla, and chocolate.

2. MCT oil capsules have the MCT oil in capsule form to help you keep in ketosis. I call these MCT oil capsules "keto on the go." (1000 milligrams per capsule)

3. High Potency Turmeric

4. Hormone Zone—nutrients including DIM that support healthy hormone levels in men and women

5. Thyroid Zone—nutrients that support healthy thyroid function

6. Fiber Zone: great-tasting psyllium husk powder with prebiotics (inulin), available flavors: berry or unflavored (contains soluble and insoluble fibers)

7. Wild Alaskan Salmon Oil

8. Enhanced Multivitamin. Enhanced multivitamins contain the active forms of vitamins, including B vitamins, with chelated minerals for better absorption of the minerals.

9. Green Supremefood: a whole food nutritional powder with fermented grasses and vegetables

10. Red Supremefood: a whole food nutritional powder with antiaging fruits

11. Ketozone Hydrolyzed collagen (vanilla and chocolate). Hydrolyzed Collagen consists of chicken collagen, containing Type I and Type II collagen. As you age, your body slowly loses collagen throughout the body (hair, nails, joints, bones, heart, and skin). Your body's joints and skin repair at night, so it's best to take ½ to 1 scoop in any liquid thirty mins before bed.

12. Divine Health Biotic: a powerful probiotic to help restore a leaky gut; contains *Bifidobacterium breve, Bifidobacterium lactis,* and *Lactobacillus plantarum.* Bacillus coagulans, and fructooligosaccharides (FOS) and galactooligosaccharides (GOS).

13. Ketosis strips

14. Fat-Zyme is a digestive enzyme designed to break down fats and vegetables and is especially helpful for patients on a Keto diet.

15. Brain Zone Basic includes the active forms of the B vitamins, curcumin, and TMG (trimethyl glycine) to lower homocysteine levels.

16. Brain Zone Advanced—a combination of nutritionals that boost BDNF (brain-derived neurotrophic factor) and NGF (neuro growth factor). These include 7,8 Dihydroxyflavone, Lion's Mane mushroom, Lithium orotate, citicoline, and tyrosine.

17. Brain Zone Focus—powdered nutritionals that energize and fuel the brain. It contains D-ribose, alpha-GPC, taurine, N-acetyl tyrosine, green tea extract, and other nutrients to help one focus and energize the brain.

18. Cellgevity—my favorite glutathione-boosting supplement (To order, call 801-316-6380, code #231599.)

To book an appointment with Dr. Colbert, call (407) 331-7007. Follow him on YouTube at Dr. Don Colbert M.D., and tune into his podcast, *Divine Health with Dr. Don Colbert,* on the Charisma Podcast Network.

A PERSONAL NOTE FROM DON COLBERT, MD

GOD DESIRES TO heal you of disease. His Word is full of promises that confirm His love for you and His desire to give you His abundant life. His desire includes more than physical health for you; He wants to make you whole in your mind and spirit as well as through a personal relationship with His Son, Jesus Christ.

If you haven't met my best friend, Jesus, I would like to take this opportunity to introduce Him to you. It is very simple. If you are ready to let Him come into your life and become your best friend, all you need to do is sincerely pray this prayer:

> *Lord Jesus, I want to know You as my Savior and Lord. I believe You are the Son of God and that You died for my sins. I also believe You were raised from the dead and now sit at the right hand of the Father praying for me. I ask You to forgive me for my sins and change my heart so that I can be Your child and live with You eternally. Thank You for Your peace. Help me to walk with You so that I can begin to know You as my best friend and my Lord. Amen.*

If you have prayed this prayer, you have just made the most important decision of your life. I rejoice with you in your decision and your new relationship with Jesus. Please contact my publisher at pray4me@charismamedia.com so that we can send you some materials that will help you become established in your relationship with the Lord. We look forward to hearing from you.

NOTES

Chapter 1

1. Ashleigh L. May et al., "Obesity—United States, 1999–2010," *Morbidity and Mortality Weekly Report* 62, no. 3 (November 22, 2013): 120–128, https://www.cdc.gov/mmwr/preview/mmwrhtml/su6203a20.htm; "Adult Obesity Facts," Centers for Disease Control and Prevention, accessed August 4, 2022, https://www.cdc.gov/obesity/data/adult.html.
2. Adekunle Sanyaolu et al., "Childhood and Adolescent Obesity in the United States: A Public Health Concern," *Global Pediatric Health* 6 (2019), https://doi.org/10.1177%2F2333794X19891305.
3. "Long-Term Trends in Diabetes," Centers for Disease Control and Prevention, April 2017, https://www.cdc.gov/diabetes/statistics/slides/long_term_trends.pdf.
4. "New CDC Report: More Than 100 Million Americans Have Diabetes or Prediabetes," Centers for Disease Control and Prevention, press release, July 18, 2017, https://www.cdc.gov/media/releases/2017/p0718-diabetes-report.html.
5. Dale E. Bredesen, MD, *The End of Alzheimer's Program* (New York: Avery, 2020), 48.
6. Ky Forward, "Women Have Double Men's Chances to Get Dementia," Women's Brain Health Initiative, accessed August 4, 2022, https://womensbrainhealth.org/think-tank/think-twice/women-have-double-mens-chances-to-get-dementia.
7. "Dementia: Number of People Affected to Triple in Next 30 Years," World Health Organization, press release, December 7, 2017, https://www.who.int/news/item/07-12-2017-dementia-number-of-people-affected-to-triple-in-next-30-years.

Chapter 2

1. Hyun Duk Yang et al., "History of Alzheimer's Disease," *Dementia and Neurocognitive Disorders* 15, no. 4 (December 2016): 115–121, https://doi.org/10.12779%2Fdnd.2016.15.4.115.
2. Yang et al., "History of Alzheimer's Disease."
3. Yang et al., "History of Alzheimer's Disease."
4. Bredesen, *The End of Alzheimer's Program*, 29–31.

5. Anna Jones, "UAB Researchers Find That 40 Percent of Young American Adults Have Insulin Resistance and Cardiovascular Risk Factors," The University of Alabama at Birmingham, September 20, 2021, https://www.uab.edu/news/research/item/12289-uab-researchers-find-that-40-percent-of-young-american-adults-have-insulin-resistance-and-cardiovascular-risk-factors.
6. Dale E. Bredesen, The End of Alzheimer's (New York: Avery, 2017), 102; Bredesen, *The End of Alzheimer's Program*, 29.
7. Bredesen, *The End of Alzheimer's*, 102–103; Bredesen, *The End of Alzheimer's Program*, 29.
8. Bredesen, The End of Alzheimer's Program, 17–18.
9. "Cardiovascular Disease Burden, Deaths Are Rising Around the World," American College of Cardiology, news release, December 9, 2020, https://www.acc.org/about-acc/press-releases/2020/12/09/18/30/cvd-burden-and-deaths-rising-around-the-world.
10. N. Nathoo et al., "Genetic Vulnerability Following Traumatic Brain Injury: The Role of Apolipoprotein E," *Molecular Pathology* 56, no. 3 (June 2003): 132–136, https://doi.org/10.1136%2Fmp.56.3.132.
11. Bredesen, *The End of Alzheimer's*, 13.

Chapter 3

1. Sanjay Gupta, *Keep Sharp* (New York: Simon & Shuster, 2021), 69.
2. "Stages of Alzheimer's Disease," Alzheimer's Association, 2018, https://www.alz.org/media/documents/alzheimers-stages-early-middle-late-ts.pdf.
3. "About Us," MoCA Cognitive Assessment, accessed August 9, 2022, https://www.mocatest.org/about/.
4. Charles Marcus et al., "Brain PET in the Diagnosis of Alzheimer's Disease," *Clinical Nuclear Medicine* 39, no.10 (October 2014): e413–e426, https://doi.org/10.1097%2FRLU.0000000000000547.

Chapter 4

1. Heidi Godman, "A Brief History of Alzheimer's Disease," Healthline, updated November 30, 2017, https://www.healthline.com/health/alzheimers-history.
2. "New Alzheimer's Association Report Reveals Sharp Increases in Alzheimer's Prevalence, Deaths, Cost of Care," Alzheimer's Association,

news release, May 30, 2018, https://www.alz.org/news/2018/new_alzheimer_s_association_report_reveals_sharp_i.

3. "What Causes Alzheimer's Disease?," National Institute on Aging, accessed August 9, 2022, https://www.nia.nih.gov/health/what-causes-alzheimers-disease#.
4. Gary Small and Gigi Vorgan, *The Memory Bible* (New York: Hachette Go, 2021), 21.
5. Bredesen, *The End of Alzheimer's Program*, 81.
6. Small and Vorgan, *The Memory Bible*, 137.
7. Minna Rusanen et al., "Heavy Smoking in Midlife and Long-Term Risk of Alzheimer Disease and Vascular Dementia," *Archives of Internal Medicine* 171, no. 4 (February 28, 2011): 333–339, https://doi.org/10.1001/archinternmed.2010.393.
8. Bredesen, *The End of Alzheimer's Program*, 17–18.
9. Bredesen, *The End of Alzheimer's Program*, 14–16.
10. Small and Vorgan, *The Memory Bible*, 265.
11. Small and Vorgan, *The Memory Bible*, 158.

Chapter 5

1. Dave Larson, "ApoE Genetics: What Your Genes Want You to Know," Life Wellness Institute, April 12, 2018, https://mylwi.com/2018/0'4/12/apoe-genetics-what-your-genes-want-you-to-know/.
2. Grzegorz Sienski et al., "APOE4 Disrupts Intracellular Lipid Homeostasis in Human iPSC-Derived Glia," *Science Translational Medicine* 13, no. 583 (March 3, 2021): 4564, https://doi.org/10.1126%2Fscitranslmed.aaz4564.
3. Gupta, *Keep Sharp*, 37.
4. Bredesen, *The End of Alzheimer's Program*, 16–17.
5. Bredesen, *The End of Alzheimer's*, 101.
6. Small and Vorgan, *The Memory Bible*, 27.
7. Small and Vorgan, *The Memory Bible*, 172–173.
8. Small and Vorgan, *The Memory Bible*, 180.
9. Bredesen, *The End of Alzheimer's Program*, 116.
10. Small and Vorgan, *The Memory Bible*, 139.

11. Joanna Lyford, “Statins Reduce Dementia Risk by 70%,” *Current Controlled Trials in Cardiovascular Medicine* 2, no. 72150 (2000), https://trialsjournal.biomedcentral.com/articles/10.1186/cvm-2001-72150.
12. Small and Vorgan, *The Memory Bible*, 180.
13. Larson, “ApoE Genetics.”
14. Bredesen, *The End of Alzheimer’s Program*, 73.
15. Brian Downer et al., “The Relationship Between Midlife and Late Life Alcohol Consumption, APOE e4 and the Decline in Learning and Memory Among Older Adults,” *Alcohol and Alcoholism* 49, no. 1 (January 2014): 17–22, https://doi.org/10.1093%2Falcalc%2Fagt144.
16. Steven Masley, *The Mediterranean Method* (New York: Harmony Books, 2019), 26.
17. “2022 Alzheimer’s Disease Facts and Figures,” Alzheimer’s Association, 2022, https://www.alz.org/media/documents/alzheimers-facts-and-figures.pdf.
18. Small and Vorgan, *The Memory Bible*, 25.

Chapter 6

1. Joseph Pizzorno, *The Toxin Solution* (New York: HarperOne, 2017), 19.
2. Neil Nathan, *Toxic* (Las Vegas, NV: Victory Belt Publishing, 2018), 25.
3. “Myths,” Alzheimer’s Association, accessed September 22, 2022, https://www.alz.org/alzheimers-dementia/what-is-alzheimers/myths.
4. Robert Siblerud et al., “A Hypothesis and Evidence That Mercury May Be an Etiological Factor in Alzheimer’s Disease,” *International Journal of Environmental Research and Public Health* 16, no. 24 (December 17, 2019): 5152, https://doi.org/10.3390/ijerph16245152.
5. Kanwal Rehman et al., “Prevalence of Exposure of Heavy Metals and Their Impact on Health Consequences,” *Journal of Cellular Biochemistry* 119, no. 1 (January 2018): 157–184, https://doi.org/10.1002/jcb.26234.
6. Zi Yang et al., “A Review on Reverse Osmosis and Nanofiltration Membranes for Water Purification,” *Polymers (Basel)* 11, no. 8 (July 29, 2019): 1252, https://doi.org/10.3390/polym11081252.
7. “Health Risks of Heavy Metals From Long-Range Transboundary Air-Pollution,” World Health Organization, 2007, https://www.who.int/publications/i/item/9789289071796.
8. Pizzorno, *The Toxin Solution*, 25.

9. Graham N. George et al., "The Chemical Forms of Mercury in Aged and Fresh Dental Amalgam Surfaces," *Chemical Research in Toxicology* 22, no. 11 (November 2009): 1761–1764, https://doi.org/10.1021%2Ftx900309c.
10. Paul E. Drevnick et al., "Increase in Mercury in Pacific Yellowfin Tuna," *Environmental Toxicology and Chemistry* 34, no. 4 (April 2015): 931–934, https://doi.org/10.1002/etc.2883.
11. "Mercury Poisoning Linked to Skin Products," US Food and Drug Administration, November 23, 2021, https://www.fda.gov/consumers/consumer-updates/mercury-poisoning-linked-skin-products.
12. Tetsuya Takahashi et al., "Methylmercury Causes Blood-Brain Barrier Damage in Rats via Upregulation of Vascular Endothelial Growth Factor Expression," *PLoS One* 12, no. 1 (January 24, 2017): e0170623, https://doi.org/10.1371/journal.pone.0170623.
13. James P. K. Rooney, "The Retention Time of Inorganic Mercury in the Brain—a Systematic Review of the Evidence," *Toxicology and Applied Pharmacology* 274, no. 3 (February 1, 2014): 425–435, https://doi.org/10.1016/j.taap.2013.12.011.
14. Jon Johnson, "Mercury Poisoning: Symptoms and Treatment," Medical News Today, January 9, 2018, https://www.medicalnewstoday.com/articles/320563.
15. Christina R. Tyler and Andrea M. Allan, "The Effects of Arsenic Exposure on Neurological and Cognitive Dysfunction in Human and Rodent Studies: A Review," *Current Environmental Health Reports* 1, no. 2 (2014): 132–147, https://doi.org/10.1007%2Fs40572-014-0012-1.
16. Benoit I. Giasson et al., "The Environmental Toxin Arsenite Induces Tau Hyperphosphorylation," *Biochemistry* 41, no. 51 (December 24, 2002): 15376–15387, https://doi.org/10.1021/bi026813c.
17. Michael Paddock, "What Is Arsenic Poisoning?," Medical News Today, January 4, 2018, https://www.medicalnewstoday.com/articles/241860.
18. Tyler and Allan, "The Effects of Arsenic Exposure on Neurological and Cognitive Dysfunction in Human and Rodent Studies."
19. Tyler and Allan, "The Effects of Arsenic Exposure on Neurological and Cognitive Dysfunction in Human and Rodent Studies."
20. Denise Wilson, "Arsenic Consumption in the United States," Western Oregon University, 2015, https://people.wou.edu/~taylors/es420_med_geo/med_geo/Wilson_2015_Arsenic_Consumption_US.pdf.
21. Sid E. O'Bryant, "Long-Term Low-Level Arsenic Exposure Is Associated With Poorer Neuropsychological Functioning: A Project FRONTIER

Study," *International Journal of Environmental Research and Public Health* 8, no. 3 (March 2011): 861–874, https://doi.org/10.3390/ijerph8030861.

22. Small and Vorgan, *The Memory Bible*, 13.
23. Siblerud et al., "A Hypothesis and Evidence That Mercury May Be an Etiological Factor in Alzheimer's Disease."
24. Daniela Ramírez Ortega et al., "Cognitive Impairment Induced by Lead Exposure During Lifespan: Mechanisms of Lead Neurotoxicity," *Toxics* 9, no. 2 (February 2021): 23, https://doi.org/10.3390%2Ftoxics9020023.
25. "Toxicological Profile for Lead," Agency for Toxic Substances and Disease Registry, Centers for Disease Control and Prevention, August 2020, https://www.atsdr.cdc.gov/toxprofiles/tp13.pdf.
26. "Lead Poisoning," Mayo Clinic, accessed August 11, 2022, https://www.mayoclinic.org/diseases-conditions/lead-poisoning/symptoms-causes/syc-20354717.
27. Pizzorno, *The Toxin Solution*, 52.
28. Daniela Ramírez Ortega et al., "Cognitive Impairment Induced by Lead Exposure During Lifespan."
29. Jong-Joo Kim et al., "Heavy Metal Toxicity: An Update of Chelating Therapeutic Strategies," *Journal of Trace Elements in Medicine and Biology* 54 (July 2019): 226–231, https://doi.org/10.1016/j.jtemb.2019.05.003.
30. Aaron Reuben, "Childhood Lead Exposure and Adult Neurodegenerative Disease," *Journal of Alzheimer's Disease* 64, no.1 (2018): 17–42, https://doi.org/10.3233%2FJAD-180267.
31. Ab Latif Wani et al., "Lead Toxicity: A Review," *Interdisciplinary Toxicology* 8, no. 2 (June 2015): 55–64, https://doi.org/10.1515%2Fintox-2015-0009.
32. "Blood Lead Reference Value," Centers for Disease Control and Prevention, last reviewed October 27, 2021, https://www.cdc.gov/nceh/lead/data/blood-lead-reference-value.htm.
33. Shaista Qadir et al., "Modulation of Plant Growth and Metabolism in Cadmium-Enriched Environments," *Reviews of Environmental Contamination and Toxicology* 229 (2014): 51–88, https://doi.org/10.1007/978-3-319-03777-6_4.
34. Agneta Åkesson et al., "Cadmium-Induced Effects on Bone in a Population-Based Study of Women," *Environmental Health Perspectives* 114, no. 6 (June 2006): 830–834, https://doi.org/10.1289%2Fehp.8763.

35. Rodjana Chunhabundit, "Cadmium Exposure and Potential Health Risk From Foods in Contaminated Area, Thailand," *Toxicological Research* 32, no. 1 (January 2016): 65–72, https://doi.org/10.5487%2FTR.2016.32.1.065.
36. Christopher D. Syme and John H. Viles, "Solution 1H NMR Investigation of Zn2+ and Cd2+ Binding to Amyloid-Beta Peptide (Abeta) of Alzheimer's Disease," *Biochimica et Biophysica Acta* 1764, no. 2 (February 2006): 246–256, https://doi.org/10.1016/j.bbapap.2005.09.012.
37. Koustav Ganguly et al., "Cadmium in Tobacco Smokers: A Neglected Link to Lung Disease?," *European Respiratory Review* 27, no. 147 (March 28, 2018): 170122, https://doi.org/10.1183/16000617.0122-2017.
38. M. Hutton, "Sources of Cadmium in the Environment," *Ecotoxicology and Environmental Safety* 7, no. 1 (February 1983): 9–24, https://doi.org/10.1016/0147-6513(83)90044-1.
39. Pizzorno, *The Toxin Solution*, 90.

Chapter 7

1. Neil Nathan, *Toxic* (Las Vegas, NV: Victory Belt Publishing, 2018), 38.
2. "About Lyme Disease Co-Infections," LymeDisease.org, accessed August 11, 2022, https://www.lymedisease.org/lyme-basics/co-infections/about-co-infections.
3. Bredesen, *The End of Alzheimer's*, 152.
4. Nathan, *Toxic*, 45, 47.
5. Nathan, *Toxic*, 26.
6. Nathan, *Toxic*, 49.
7. "Lab Tests," Surviving Mold, accessed August 11, 2022, https://www.survivingmold.com/resources-for-patients/diagnosis/lab-tests.
8. Nathan, *Toxic*, 50.

Chapter 8

1. Gupta, *Keep Sharp*, 237.
2. Shelly L. Gray et al., "Cumulative Use of Strong Anticholinergics and Incident Dementia," *JAMA Internal Medicine* 173, no. 3 (March 2015): 401–407, https://doi.org/10.1001/jamainternmed.2014.7663.
3. Gray et al., "Cumulative Use of Strong Anticholinergics and Incident Dementia."

Chapter 9

1. Catharine Ross et al., eds., *Modern Nutrition in Health and Disease*, 11th ed. (Burlington, MA: Jones & Bartlett Learning, 2020), ch. 12.
2. Hajo Haase and Lothar Rink, "The Immune System and the Impact of Zinc During Aging," *Immunity and Ageing* 6 (2009): 9, https://doi.org/10.1186%2F1742-4933-6-9.
3. "Copper," National Institutes of Health, updated March 29, 2021, https://ods.od.nih.gov/factsheets/Copper-HealthProfessional/.
4. Bredesen, *The End of Alzheimer's*, 132–133.
5. "Zinc," National Institutes of Health, updated August 2, 2022, https://ods.od.nih.gov/factsheets/Zinc-HealthProfessional/.
6. "Zinc," National Institutes of Health.

Chapter 10

1. Bernadene Magnuson, "Aspartame—Facts and Fiction," *New Zealand Medical Journal* 123, no. 1311 (2010): 53–7, https://pubmed.ncbi.nlm.nih.gov/20360796/.
2. Arbind Kumar Choudhary and Yeong Yeh Lee, "Neurophysiological Symptoms and Aspartame: What is the Connection?," *Nutritional Neuroscience* 21, no. 5 (June 2018): 306–316, https://doi.org/10.1080/1028415x.2017.1288340; Glenda N. Lindseth et al., "Neurobehavioral Effects of Aspartame Consumption," *Research in Nursing & Health* 37, no. 3 (June 2014): 185–193, https://doi.org/10.1002%2Fnur.21595.
3. "Additional Information About High-Intensity Sweeteners Permitted for Use in Food in the United States," US Food and Drug Administration, February 8, 2018, https://www.fda.gov/food/food-additives-petitions/additional-information-about-high-intensity-sweeteners-permitted-use-food-united-states#.
4. Sanchari Chattopadhyay et al., "Artificial Sweeteners—a Review," *Journal of Food Science and Technology* 51, no. 4 (April 2014): 611–621, https://doi.org/10.1007%2Fs13197-011-0571-1.
5. Kamila Czarnecka et al., "Aspartame—True or False? Narrative Review of Safety Analysis of General Use in Products," *Nutrients* 13, no. 6 (June 2021): 1957, https://doi.org/10.3390%2Fnu13061957.
6. Choudhary and Lee, "Neurophysiological Symptoms and Aspartame."
7. Richard J. Wurtman, "Neurochemical Changes Following High-Dose Aspartame With Dietary Carbohydrates [Letter]," *New England Journal*

of Medicine 309 (August 1983): 429–430, https://doi.org/10.1056/NEJM198308183090710.

8. Matthew P. Pase et al., "Sugar- and Artificially Sweetened Beverages and the Risks of Incident Stroke and Dementia: A Prospective Cohort Study," *Stroke* 48, no. 5 (May 2017): 1139–1146, https://doi.org/10.1161/strokeaha.116.016027.
9. Small and Vorgan, *The Memory Bible*, 156.
10. Bredesen, *The End of Alzheimer's*, 50.
11. Bredesen, *The End of Alzheimer's*, 51.

Chapter 11

1. Small and Vorgan, *The Memory Bible*, 186.
2. Bredesen, *The End of Alzheimer's Program*, 177–178.
3. Riki E. Slayday et al., "Interaction Between Alcohol Consumption and Apolipoprotein E (ApoE) Genotype With Cognition in Middle-Aged Men," *Journal of the International Neuropsychological Society* 27, no. 1 (January 2021): 56–68, https://doi.org/10.1017/s1355617720000570.
4. Downer et al., "The Relationship Between Midlife and Late Life Alcohol Consumption."
5. "How Does Alcohol Affect the Brain?," StoneRidge Centers, accessed August 12, 2022, https://stoneridgecenters.com/how-does-alcohol-affect-the-brain/.

Chapter 12

1. Bredesen, *The End of Alzheimer's Program*, 115.
2. Takanori Honda et al., "Serum Elaidic Acid Concentration and Risk of Dementia: The Hisayama Study," *Neurology* 93, no. 22 (November 26, 2019): e2053–e2064, https://doi.org/10.1212/wnl.0000000000008464.
3. Meagan Bridges, "Facts About Trans Fats," Medline Plus, reviewed May 26, 2020, https://medlineplus.gov/ency/patientinstructions/000786.htm.
4. E. Ginter and V. Simko, "New Data on Harmful Effects of Trans-Fatty Acids," *Bratislava Medical Journal* 117, no. 5 (2016): 251–253, https://doi.org/10.4149/bll_2016_048.
5. Bredesen, *The End of Alzheimer's Program*, 116.

Chapter 13

1. Small and Vorgan, *The Memory Bible*, 205.
2. Small and Vorgan, *The Memory Bible*, 205.
3. Bredesen, *The End of Alzheimer's Program*, 287–288.
4. Pin-Liang Chen et al., "Risk of Dementia After Anaesthesia and Surgery," *British Journal of Psychiatry* 204, no. 3 (March 2014): 188–193, https://doi.org/10.1192%2Fbjp.bp.112.119610.
5. Young-Suk Kwon et al., "Risk of Dementia in Patients Who Underwent Surgery Under Neuraxial Anesthesia: A Nationwide Cohort Study," *Journal of Personalized Medicine* 11, no. 12 (December 2021): 1386, https://doi.org/10.3390%2Fjpm11121386.
6. Small and Vorgan, *The Memory Bible*, 204.
7. "How to Reduce Cortisol and Turn Down the Dial on Stress," Cleveland Clinic, August 27, 2020, https://health.clevelandclinic.org/how-to-reduce-cortisol-and-turn-down-the-dial-on-stress/.

Chapter 14

1. Shweta Patel et al., "The Association Between Cannabis Use and Schizophrenia: Causative or Curative? A Systematic Review," *Cureus Journal of Medical Science* 12, no. 7 (July 2020): e9309, https://doi.org/10.7759%2Fcureus.9309.
2. See Shawna Seed, "Schizophrenia and Marijuana: Trigger or Treatment?," WebMD, October 20, 2020, https://www.webmd.com/schizophrenia/schizophrenia-marijuana-link; Patel et al., "The Association Between Cannabis Use and Schizophrenia"; "Is There a Link Between Marijuana Use and Psychiatric Disorders?," National Institute on Drug Abuse, April 13, 2021, https://nida.nih.gov/publications/research-reports/marijuana/there-link-between-marijuana-use-psychiatric-disorders#.
3. Small and Vorgan, *The Memory Bible*, 189.
4. Bredesen, *The End of Alzheimer's*, 50.
5. Valentina Lorenzetti et al., "Adolescent Cannabis Use, Cognition, Brain Health and Educational Outcomes: A Review of the Evidence," *European Neuropsychopharmacology* 36 (July 2020): 169–180, https://doi.org/10.1016/j.euroneuro.2020.03.012.
6. Lorenzetti et al., "Adolescent Cannabis Use."
7. Small and Vorgan, *The Memory Bible*, 188.

8. Elizabeth Stuyt, "The Problem With the Current High Potency THC Marijuana From the Perspective of an Addiction Psychiatrist," *Missouri Medicine* 115, no. 6 (November–December 2018): 482–486, https://www.ncbi.nlm.nih.gov/pmc/articles/PMC6312155/.
9. Stuyt, "The Problem With the Current High Potency THC Marijuana From the Perspective of an Addiction Psychiatrist."
10. Gary K. Hulse et al., "Dementia Associated With Alcohol and Other Drug Use," *International Psychogeriatrics* 17, supplement 1 (2005): S109–S127, https://doi.org/10.1017/s1041610205001985.
11. K. D. Ersche et al., "Cocaine Dependence: A Fast-Track for Brain Ageing?," *Molecular Psychiatry* 18 (2013): 134–135, https://doi.org/10.1038/mp.2012.31.
12. Nian-sheng Tzeng et al., "Association Between Amphetamine-Related Disorder and Dementia—a Nationwide Cohort Study in Taiwan," *Annals of Clinical and Translational Neurology* 7, no. 8 (August 2020): 1284–1295, https://doi.org/10.1002%2Facn3.51113.
13. Simon Andrew Vann Jones and Allison O'Kelly, "Psychedelics as a Treatment for Alzheimer's Disease Dementia," *Frontiers in Synaptic Neuroscience* (August 21, 2020), https://doi.org/10.3389/fnsyn.2020.00034.

Chapter 15

1. Gupta, *Keep Sharp*, 187.
2. Gupta, *Keep Sharp*, 62–65.
3. Karin Lopatko Lindman et al., "Herpesvirus Infections, Antiviral Treatment, and the Risk of Dementia—a Registry-Based Cohort Study in Sweden," *Alzheimer's and Dementia (NY)* 7, no. 1 (February 14, 2021): e12119, https://doi.org/10.1002/trc2.12119.
4. Samuel Alizon et al., "Towards a Multi-Level and a Multi-Disciplinary Approach to DNA Oncovirus Virulence," *Philosophical Transactions of the Royal Society B: Biological Sciences* 374, no. 1773 (May 27, 2019): 20190041, https://doi.org/10.1098/rstb.2019.0041.
5. Anthony N. van den Pol, "Viral Infection Leading to Brain Dysfunction: More Prevalent Than Appreciated?," *Neuron* 64, no. 1 (October 15, 2009): 17–20, https://doi.org/10.1016%2Fj.neuron.2009.09.023.

Chapter 16

1. Bredesen, *The End of Alzheimer's Program*, 70.
2. Small and Vorgan, *The Memory Bible*, 21.
3. Gupta, *Keep Sharp*, 59.
4. Gupta, *Keep Sharp*, 61.
5. Bredesen, *The End of Alzheimer's Program*, 97–98.
6. Bredesen, *The End of Alzheimer's*, 42.
7. Bredesen, *The End of Alzheimer's*, 31.
8. Small and Vorgan, *The Memory Bible*, 14.

Chapter 17

1. Will Cole, *Ketotarian* (New York: Avery, 2018), 224.
2. Bredesen, *The End of Alzheimer's Program*, 73.
3. Steven Masley, The Mediterranean Method (New York: Harmony Books, 2019), 97.
4. Small and Vorgan, *The Memory Bible*, 159.
5. Mark Hyman, *The Pegan Diet* (New York: Little, Brown Spark, 2021), 131.

Chapter 18

1. Kushagra Mathur et al., "Effect of Artificial Sweeteners on Insulin Resistance Among Type-2 Diabetes Mellitus Patients," *Journal of Family Medicine and Primary Care* 9, no. 1 (January 28, 2020): 69–71, https://doi.org/10.4103/jfmpc.jfmpc_329_19.
2. "Autointoxication—a Major Cause of Disease," Modern Manna, accessed September 18, 2022, https://www.modernmanna.org/2015/12/15/autointoxication-a-major-cause-of-disease/.
3. Pizzorno, *The Toxin Solution*, 98.
4. Margaret E. Sears et al., "Arsenic, Cadmium, Lead, and Mercury in Sweat: A Systematic Review," *Journal of Environmental and Public Health* 2012 (February 22, 2012), https://doi.org/10.1155/2012/184745.
5. Gray et al., "Cumulative Use of Strong Anticholinergics and Incident Dementia."
6. Pizzorno, *The Toxin Solution*, 123.
7. Pizzorno, *The Toxin Solution*, 52.

8. W. H. Wilson Tang et al., "Intestinal Microbial Metabolism of Phosphatidylcholine and Cardiovascular Risk," *New England Journal of Medicine* 368, no. 17 (April 25, 2013): 1575–1584, https://doi.org/10.1056/nejmoa1109400.

Chapter 19

1. "2022 Alzheimer's Disease Facts and Figures," Alzheimer's Association.
2. "Inflammation," Cleveland Clinic, accessed September 19, 2022, https://my.clevelandclinic.org/health/symptoms/21660-inflammation
3. Bredesen, *The End of Alzheimer's Program*, 20.
4. David Perlmutter with Kristin Loberg, *Brain Maker: The Power of Gut Microbes to Heal and Protect Your Brain—for Life* (New York: Little, Brown Spark, 2015), 57.
5. Pizzorno, *The Toxin Solution*, 112.
6. Robert Keith Wallace and Samantha Wallace, *Gut Crisis: How Diet, Probiotics, and Friendly Bacteria Help You Lose Weight and Heal Your Body and Mind* (Fairfield, IA: Dharma, 2017), 86–87.
7. Pizzorno, *The Toxin Solution*, 112–114, 119–120, 126.
8. Bredesen, *The End of Alzheimer's*, 45.

Chapter 20

1. Chris Kresser, "Intermittent Fasting: The Science Behind the Trend," Chris Kresser, March 25, 2019, https://chriskresser.com/intermittent-fasting-the-science-behind-the-trend/.
2. Bredesen, *The End of Alzheimer's Program*, 93.
3. Aaron Kandola, "What Are the Benefits of Intermittent Fasting?," Medical News Today, November 7, 2018, https://www.medicalnewstoday.com/articles/323605.
4. Andrea RodriguesVasconcelos et al., "Effects of Intermittent Fasting on Age-Related Changes on Na,K-ATPase Activity and Oxidative Status Induced by Lipopolysaccharide in Rat Hippocampus," *Neurobiology of Aging* 36, no. 5 (May 2014): 1914-1923, https://doi.org/10.1016/j.neurobiolaging.2015.02.020.
5. Kandola, "What Are the Benefits of Intermittent Fasting?"
6. Kresser, "Intermittent Fasting."
7. Kandola, "What Are the Benefits of Intermittent Fasting?"

8. Mark P. Mattson et al., "Intermittent Metabolic Switching, Neuroplasticity and Brain Health," *Nature Review Neuroscience* 19, no. 2 (February 2018): 63–80, https://doi.org/10.1038%2Fnrn.2017.156.
9. Kresser, "Intermittent Fasting."
10. Joe Sugarman, "Are There Any Proven Benefits to Fasting?," Johns Hopkins Health Review, archived April 16, 2018, https://web.archive.org/web/20160418032921/https://www.johnshopkinshealthreview.com/issues/spring-summer-2016/articles/are-there-any-proven-benefits-to-fasting.

Chapter 21

1. Shalini Paruthi et al., "Recommended Amount of Sleep for Pediatric Populations: A Consensus Statement of the American Academy of Sleep Medicine," *Journal of Clinical Sleep Medicine* 12, no. 6 (June 15, 2016): 785–786, https://doi.org/10.5664%2Fjcsm.5866; Anne G. Wheaton et al., "Sleep Duration and Injury-Related Risk Behaviors Among High School Students—United States, 2007–2013," *Morbidity and Mortality Weekly Report* 65, no. 13 (April 8, 2016): 337–341, http://dx.doi.org/10.15585/mmwr.mm6513a1.
2. Jeffrey M. Jones, "In U.S., 40% Get Less Than Recommended Amount of Sleep," Gallup, December 19, 2013, https://news.gallup.com/poll/166553/less-recommended-amount-sleep.aspx.
3. [3] Wendy Myers, "Complete List of Artificial Sweeteners," Myers Detox, accessed August 14, 2022, https://myersdetox.com/complete-list-of-artificial-sweeteners/.
4. Hyman, *The Pegan Diet*, 93.
5. Bredesen, *The End of Alzheimer's Program*, 45.
6. Gupta, *Keep Sharp*, 137.
7. Bredesen, *The End of Alzheimer's Program*, 214.
8. Gupta, *Keep Sharp*, 140–141.
9. Bredesen, *The End of Alzheimer's Program*, 214.
10. "Sleep and Sleep Disorder Statistics," American Sleep Association, accessed August 14, 2022, https://www.sleepassociation.org/about-sleep/sleep-statistics/.
11. Deidre Conroy, "3 Reasons Women Are More Likely to Have Insomnia," Michigan Health, June 13, 2016, https://healthblog.uofmhealth.org/health-management/3-reasons-women-are-more-likely-to-have-insomnia.
12. Bredesen, *The End of Alzheimer's Program*, 217.

13. Elaine Finucane et al., "Does Reading a Book in Bed Make a Difference to Sleep in Comparison to Not Reading a Book in Bed? The People's Trial—an Online, Pragmatic, Randomised Trial," *Trials* 22, no. 873 (2021), https://doi.org/10.1186/s13063-021-05831-3.
14. Bredesen, *The End of Alzheimer's Program*, 222.

CHAPTER 22

1. Robert M. Sapolsky, *Why Zebras Don't Get Ulcers*, 3rd edition (New York: Henry Holt and Company, 2004), 210.
2. Sapolsky, *Why Zebras Don't Get Ulcers*, 213.
3. Bredesen, *The End of Alzheimer's Program*, 228.
4. Small and Vorgan, *The Memory Bible*, 58.
5. Gupta, *Keep Sharp*, 108.
6. Sapolsky, *Why Zebras Don't Get Ulcers*, 215–219.
7. Cole, *Ketotarian*, 15.
8. Healthline, "Five Ways Reading Can Improve Health and Well-Being," HuffPost, updated October 13, 2017, https://www.huffpost.com/entry/five-ways-reading-can-imp_b_12456962.
9. Small and Vorgan, *The Memory Bible*, 69.
10. See the work of Earl K. Miller and the Miller Lab: http://millerlab.mit.edu.
11. Small and Vorgan, *The Memory Bible*, 60–61.

CHAPTER 23

1. Gupta, *Keep Sharp*, 101.
2. Bredesen, *The End of Alzheimer's Program*, 200.
3. "Table 25. Participation in Leisure-Time Aerobic and Muscle-Strengthening Activities That Meet the Federal 2008 Physical Activity Guidelines for Americans Among Adults Aged 18 and Over, by Selected Characteristics: United States, Selected Years 1998–2018," Centers for Disease Control and Prevention, 2019, https://www.cdc.gov/nchs/data/hus/2019/025-508.pdf.
4. Thom Rieck, "10,000 Steps a Day: Too Low? Too high?," Mayo Clinic, March 23, 2020, https://www.mayoclinic.org/healthy-lifestyle/fitness/in-depth/10000-steps/art-20317391#.
5. Small and Vorgan, *The Memory Bible*, 175.

6. Bredesen, *The End of Alzheimer's Program*, 201.
7. Small and Vorgan, *The Memory Bible*, 173.
8. Peter Elwood et al., "Healthy Lifestyles Reduce the Incidence of Chronic Diseases and Dementia: Evidence From the Caerphilly Cohort Study," *PLoS One* 8, no. 12 (December 9, 2013): e81877, https://doi.org/10.1371/journal.pone.0081877.
9. Bredesen, *The End of Alzheimer's Program*, 203.
10. David C. Peritz et al., "The Role of Stress Testing in the Older Athlete," American College of Cardiology, November 6, 2017, https://www.acc.org/latest-in-cardiology/articles/2017/11/06/10/32/the-role-of-stress-testing-in-the-older-athlete#.
11. "Coronary Artery Disease—Coronary Heart Disease," American Heart Association, accessed October 20, 2022, https://www.heart.org/en/health-topics/consumer-healthcare/what-is-cardiovascular-disease/coronary-artery-disease.
12. Phillip Nieto, "Cognitive Decline Can Be Avoided With Simple Everyday Exercises, New Study Suggests," Fox News, August 3, 2022, https://www.foxnews.com/health/cognitive-decline-avoided-simple-everday-exercises-new-study-suggests.
13. Pedro F. Saint-Maurice et al., "Association of Leisure-Time Physical Activity Across the Adult Life Course With All-Cause and Cause-Specific Mortality," *JAMA Network Open* 2, no. 3 (March 1, 2019): e190355, https://doi.org/10.1001/jamanetworkopen.2019.0355.

Chapter 24

1. Y. Handa et al., "Estrogen Concentrations in Beef and Human Hormone-Dependent Cancers," *Annals of Oncology* 20, no. 9 (September 1, 2009): 1610–1611, https://doi.org/10.1093/annonc/mdp381.
2. "Early Menopause May Raise Risk of Dementia Later in Life," American Heart Association, March 1, 2022, https://newsroom.heart.org/news/early-menopause-may-raise-risk-of-dementia-later-in-life.
3. Robert Hart, "Viagra Use May Reduce Risk of Getting Alzheimer's by Nearly 70%, Study Suggests," *Forbes*, updated April 21, 2022, https://www.forbes.com/sites/roberthart/2021/12/06/viagra-use-may-reduce-risk-of-getting-alzheimers-by-nearly-70-study-suggests/?sh=7159d673ad72.
4. Bredesen, *The End of Alzheimer's*, 131.
5. Bredesen, *The End of Alzheimer's*, 131.

6. Erica Zelfand, "Pregnenolone for Memory, Mood, and Brain Health," Allergy Research Group, 2019, https://www.allergyresearchgroup.com/blog/pregnenolone-and-memory.
7. Thomas Guilliams, "Re-assessing the Notion of 'Pregnenolone Steal,'" *ZRT Blog*, June 21, 2017, https://www.zrtlab.com/blog/archive/reassessing-pregnenolone-steal.
8. "Breast Cancer in Young Women," Centers for Disease Control and Prevention, accessed September 20, 2022, https://www.cdc.gov/cancer/breast/young_women/bringyourbrave/breast_cancer_young_women/index.htm#:~:text=Breast%20cancer%20is%20the%20most,under%20the%20age%20of%2045.
9. Bredesen, *The End of Alzheimer's*, 51.
10. Anna-Karin Lennartsson et al., "Perceived Stress at Work Is Associated With Lower Levels of DHEA-S," *PLoS One* 8, no. 8 (2013): e72460, https://doi.org/10.1371%2Fjournal.pone.0072460.
11. Small and Vorgan, *The Memory Bible*, 175.
12. Avrum Bluming and Carol Tavris, *Estrogen Matters* (New York: Little, Brown Spark, 2018), 237.
13. Marianne Thvilum et al., "Increased Risk of Dementia in Hypothyroidism: A Danish Nationwide Register-Based Study," *Clinical Endocrinology* 94, no. 6 (June 2021): 1017–1024, https://doi.org/10.1111/cen.14424.
14. Peter Celec et al., "On the Effects of Testosterone on Brain Behavioral Functions," *Frontiers in Neuroscience* 9 (2015), https://doi.org/10.3389/fnins.2015.00012.
15. D. A. Rivas and R. A. Fielding, "Exercise as a Countermeasure for Sarcopenia," in *Sarcopenia—Age-Related Muscle Wasting and Weakness*, ed. Gordon S. Lynch (New York: Springer, 2011), 334.
16. "Low Testosterone," American Diabetes Association, archived July 15, 2019, https://web.archive.org/web/20190715194104/http://www.diabetes.org/living-with-diabetes/treatment-and-care/men/low-testosterone.html.

Chapter 25

1. Bredesen, *The End of Alzheimer's*, 8.
2. "Aricept Side Effects," Drugs.com, updated April 29, 2022, https://www.drugs.com/sfx/aricept-side-effects.html.
3. Small and Vorgan, *The Memory Bible*, 163.
4. Small and Vorgan, *The Memory Bible*, 164.

5. Gupta, *Keep Sharp*, 161.
6. Bredesen, *The End of Alzheimer's*, 179.
7. Oliver E. Owen and Richard W. Hanson, "Ketone Bodies," Science Direct, accessed September 13, 2021, https://www.sciencedirect.com/topics/neuroscience/ketone-bodies.
8. Matthew K. Taylor et al., "Feasibility and Efficacy Data From a Ketogenic Diet Intervention in Alzheimer's Disease," *Alzheimer's & Dementia (NY)* 4 (2018): 28–36, https://doi.org/10.1016%2Fj.trci.2017.11.002.
9. T. B. Vanitallie et al., "Treatment of Parkinson Disease With Diet-Induced Hyperketonemia: A Feasibility Study," *Neurology* 64, no. 4 (February 22, 2005): 728–730, https://doi.org/10.1212/01.wnl.0000152046.11390.45.
10. Bredesen, *The End of Alzheimer's Program*, 74.
11. Josh Axe, *Keto Diet* (New York: Little, Brown Spark, 2019), 116.

Chapter 26

1. Bredesen, *The End of Alzheimer's Program*, 114.
2. Bredesen, *The End of Alzheimer's Program*, 122.
3. Bredesen, *The End of Alzheimer's Program*, 302–303.
4. Gupta, *Keep Sharp*, 88.
5. Bredesen, *The End of Alzheimer's Program*, 154–155.
6. Freydis Hjalmarsdottir, "How Much Omega-3 Should You Take per Day?," Healthline, December 15, 2019, https://www.healthline.com/nutrition/how-much-omega-3.
7. Yuusuke Saitsu et al., "Improvement of Cognitive Functions by Oral Intake of Hericium Erinaceus," *Biomedical Research* 40, no. 4 (2019): 125–131, https://doi.org/10.2220/biomedres.40.125.
8. Bredesen, *The End of Alzheimer's Program*, 135.
9. Small and Vorgan, *The Memory Bible*, 149.
10. Susan J. Hewlings and Douglas S. Kalman, "Curcumin: A Review of Its Effects on Human Health," *Foods* 6, no. 10 (2017): 92, https://doi.org/10.3390/foods6100092.
11. Gary W. Small et al., "Memory and Brain Amyloid and Tau Effects of a Bioavailable Form of Curcumin in Non-Demented Adults: A Double-Blind, Placebo-Controlled 18-Month Trial," *American Journal of*

Geriatric Psychiatry 26, no. 3 (March 1, 2018): P266–P277, https://doi.org/10.1016/j.jagp.2017.10.010.

12. Bredesen, *The End of Alzheimer's Program*, 183.
13. Bredesen, *The End of Alzheimer's*, 103.
14. Bredesen, *The End of Alzheimer's*, 199–121.
15. Traci Stein, "A Genetic Mutation That Can Affect Mental & Physical Health," *Psychology Today*, September 5, 2014, https://www.psychologytoday.com/us/blog/the-integrationist/201409/genetic-mutation-can-affect-mental-physical-health.
16. Ronald Grisanti, "SMASH: The Potent Recipe for Increasing Omega 3," Functional Medicine University, accessed August 14, 2022, https://www.functionalmedicineuniversity.com/public/1718.cfm.
17. Jim Kwik, *Limitless* (Carlsbad, CA: Hay House, 2020), 38.
18. Pizzorno, *The Toxin Solution*, 112–114, 119–120, 126.
19. Bredesen, *The End of Alzheimer's Program*, 156.
20. Small and Vorgan, *The Memory Bible*, 143.
21. Small and Vorgan, *The Memory Bible*, 154–155.
22. Bredesen, *The End of Alzheimer's Program*, 12.
23. Bredesen, *The End of Alzheimer's Program*, 200.
24. Alessandra Berry et al., "NGF, Brain and Behavioral Plasticity," *Neural Plasticity* (2012): 784040, https://doi.org/10.1155%2F2012%2F784040.
25. Small and Vorgan, *The Memory Bible*, 153.
26. Anthony G. Pacholko and Lane K. Bekar, "Lithium Orotate: A Superior Option for Lithium Therapy?," *Brain and Behavior* 11, no. 8 (August 2021): e2262, https://doi.org/10.1002%2Fbrb3.2262.
27. Lars Vedel Kessing et al., "Association of Lithium in Drinking Water With the Incidence of Dementia," *JAMA Psychiatry* 74, no. 10 (2017): 1005–1010, https://doi.org/10.1001/jamapsychiatry.2017.2362.
28. Young-Sung Kim et al., "Neuroprotective Effects of Magnesium L-Threonate in a Hypoxic Zebrafish Model," *BMC Neuroscience* 21, no. 1 (June 26, 2020): 29, https://doi.org/10.1186/s12868-020-00580-6; Aparna Ann Mathew and Rajitha Panonnummal, "'Magnesium'—the Master Cation—as a Drug—Possibilities and Evidences," *Biometals* 34, no. 5 (2021): 955–986, https://doi.org/10.1007%2Fs10534-021-00328-7.

Chapter 27

1. Robert S. Wilson et al., "Life-Span Cognitive Activity, Neuropathologic Burden, and Cognitive Aging," *Neurology* 81, no. 4 (July 23, 2013): 314–321, https://doi.org/10.1212%2FWNL.0b013e31829c5e8a.
2. Cristy Phillips, "Lifestyle Modulators of Neuroplasticity: How Physical Activity, Mental Engagement, and Diet Promote Cognitive Health During Aging," *Neural Plasticity* (2017), https://doi.org/10.1155/2017/3589271.
3. Snorri Bjorn Rafnsson et al., "Loneliness, Social Integration, and Incident Dementia Over 6 Years: Prospective Findings From the English Longitudinal Study of Ageing," *Journals of Gerontology* 75, no. 1 (January 2020): 114–124, https://doi.org/10.1093/geronb/gbx087.
4. Small and Vorgan, *The Memory Bible*, 190–191.
5. Gupta, *Keep Sharp*, 43.
6. Gupta, *Keep Sharp*, 44.
7. Small and Vorgan, *The Memory Bible*, 17.
8. Gupta, *Keep Sharp*, 44.
9. Small and Vorgan, *The Memory Bible*, 85.
10. Gupta, *Keep Sharp*, 68.
11. Kwik, *Limitless*, 47.
12. Small and Vorgan, *The Memory Bible*, 93.
13. Small and Vorgan, *The Memory Bible*, 13.

Chapter 28

1. Bredesen, *The End of Alzheimer's*, 26.
2. Gupta, *Keep Sharp*, 63.

INDEX

P

R

S

T

U

V

W

MY **FREE GIFT** TO YOU

Thank you for reading *Dr. Colbert's Healthy Brain Zone*. I hope you now feel equipped with the tools and knowledge you need to prevent, slow, and fight off cognitive disorders like dementia and Alzheimer's disease. I pray this book helps add vitality and life for your years still to come.

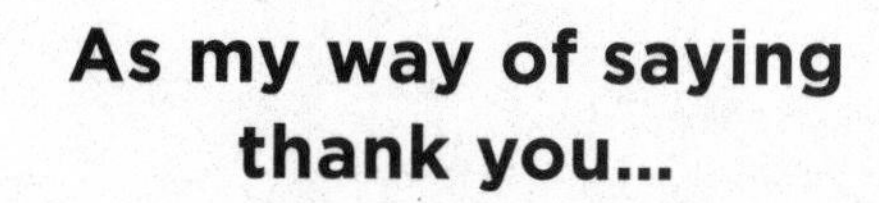

As my way of saying thank you...

I am offering you the *Dr. Colbert's Healthy Gut Zone* e-book for FREE!

To get this free gift, please go to DrColbertBooks.com/gift2023

Thank you, and God bless,

Dr. Don Colbert

SILOAM